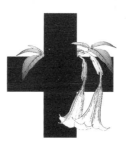

# Poisonous Plants of Paradise

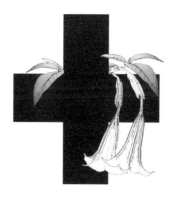

# Poisonous Plants of Paradise

## First Aid and Medical Treatment of Injuries from Hawai'i's Plants

Susan Scott
and
Craig Thomas, M.D.

*A Latitude 20 Book*

UNIVERSITY OF HAWAI'I PRESS

Honolulu

00  01  02  03  04  05      5  4  3  2  1

**Library of Congress Cataloging-in-Publication Data**
Scott, Susan, 1948–
Poisonous plants of paradise : first aid and medical treatment of injuries from Hawai'i's plants / Susan Scott and Craig Thomas.
p.  cm.
"A latitude 20 book."
Includes bibliographical references and index.
ISBN 0–8248–2251–X (alk. paper)
1. Poisonous plants—Hawaii—Toxicology.  2. First aid in illness and injury.
3. Antidotes.  I. Thomas, Craig, 1952–  II. Title.

RA1250 .S365  2000
615.9′52′09969—dc21                    99–050088

*Cover and book designed by Santos B. Barbasa Jr.*

*Printed through Asia Pacific Offset, Inc.*

*To Claire and Tommy Thomas.*
*Thank you for sharing your love of learning.*
*Your curiosity about the world inspires us.*

# CONTENTS

# PREFACE

The first book we wrote together, *All Stings Considered: First Aid and Medical Treatment of Hawaii's Marine Injuries,* was about medical problems associated with being in the ocean. After it was published, in 1997, we were surprised when people began asking us questions about mango rash and poinsettia poisoning. Because we did not know the answers, we decided to begin another literature search and write another book—about poisonous plants in Hawai'i.

Choosing which plants to include in this book was difficult because the list of plants potentially harmful to humans is nearly endless. We consulted the following books, using them as a basis for selecting individual species: Harry L. Arnold's 1968 *Poisonous Plants of Hawaii,* Roger Baldwin's 1979 *Hawaii's Poisonous Plants,* and Julia Morton's 1995 *Plants Poisonous to People in Florida and Other Warm Areas.* Working from that foundation, we made our decisions about whether to include a plant by evaluating its toxicity, its abundance in Hawai'i, and/or its reputation for causing medical problems.

We searched the current medical literature through Internet Grateful Med, the on-line database of the National Library of Medicine. We also looked up each topic in Micromedex Inc., a computer database of medical information designed for emergency physicians and poison control centers. These databases are excellent sources of current medical literature but contain far more detailed information than we could include here. For readers interested in learning more, we highly recommend browsing both databases.

Many of the plants discussed in this book are used in traditional and folk medicine. Because we have based our medical recommendations on literature published in peer-reviewed journals, we do not endorse unstudied treatments. Without scientific proof of their efficacy, home remedies and traditional medicines may make a condition worse or, in some cases, even cause death. For plants that are known to be used as remedies for certain ailments, we included descriptions of the remedies to help medical practitioners diagnose plant-induced illnesses that may occur from these treatments.

In writing this book, we use everyday language as often as

possible, to make the information accessible to a wide range of people. Because medical workers use unique terminology, though, we use medical nomenclature in the Advanced Medical Treatment sections.

In the First Aid sections, we have often recommended hydrocortisone cream and diphenhydramine tablets (Benadryl) to relieve symptoms of itching and mild allergy. We chose these medications because they are common, inexpensive, and available without a prescription. Similar medications—some over-the-counter, some prescription—will also relieve these symptoms and may work better for some individuals.

If a person's exposure to a plant makes an emergency room visit necessary, it is important to take a sample of the leaves, flowers, and stems with you for identification. Because professionals need more than a flower petal or piece of leaf to distinguish a species, take as much of the culprit plant with you as possible. If there is any question about the plant's toxicity to the skin, wear gloves while collecting the plant, bag it in paper or plastic, then thoroughly wash your hands.

A few of our recommendations are new and may require some getting used to. For instance, we do not recommend giving Ipecac, or inducing vomiting in any other way, as first aid for plant poisonings. Vomiting in a victim who may have altered consciousness, or who has eaten something caustic, may do more harm than good, or even cause death.

If you disagree with any of our conclusions, we urge you to check our sources and contact us. We can be reached through our publisher and will be interested to learn of new data, new incidents, or any errors we may have made.

Hawai'i hosts tropical plants from all over the world, and the Islands are packed with spectacular gardens and breathtaking landscapes. We hope that by learning which plants are potentially poisonous, you will enjoy them all the more.

# TOXIN CATEGORIES OF POISONOUS PLANTS IN HAWAI'I

*Anticholinergics*
> Angel's Trumpet
> Jimsonweed
> Lantana

*Anticholinergics plus Solanine*
> Nightshade
> Cestrum
> Cup of Gold and Silver Cup

*Calcium Oxalate Crystals*
> Anthurium
> Dumb Cane
> Elephant Ear
> Taro

*Cardiac Glycosides*
> Be-Still Tree
> Cerbera
> Crown Flower
> Foxglove
> Oleander

*Colchicine*
> Gloriosa Lily

*Cyanogenic Glycoside*
> Cassava
> Hydrangea

*Diphenyl Lobelidiol*
> Star-of-Bethlehem

## Grayanotoxins
Azalea

## Kavalactones
Kava

## Phytolaccine
Pokeberry and Coral Berry

## Protoanemonin
Japanese Anemone

## Skin and/or Stomach Irritants
Allamanda
Candlenut (*Kukui*)
Cashew
Hawaiian Poppy
Kāhili Flower
Mango
Pencil Plant, Crown of Thorns, Red Spurge,
    and Slipper Flower
Plumeria
Poinsettia
Silky Oak

## Tetranortriterpene (Neurotoxin)
Chinaberry

## Toxalbumins
Black-Eyed Susan
Castor Bean
*Jatropha* species

## Vinblastine and Vincristine
Periwinkle

### *Mushroom Toxins Found in Hawai'i* (ordered from most common poisonings to least common poisonings)

Gastrointestinal Irritants (specific toxins unknown)
Hallucinogenics (psilocybin and others)
Muscimol-Ibotenic Acid
Cyclopeptides (amatoxins)
Coprine

# FAMILIES OF POISONOUS PLANTS IN HAWAI'I

**Bellflower Family, Campanulaceae**
  Star-of-Bethlehem (*Hippobroma longiflora* [L.] G. Don)

**Buttercup Family, Ranunculaceae**
  Japanese Anemone (*Anemone hupehensis* Lemoine)

**Dogbane Family, Apocynaceae**
  Allamanda (*Allamanda cathartica* L.)
  Be-Still Tree (*Thevetia peruviana* [Pers.] Schumann)
  Cerbera (*Cerbera manghas* L.)
  Oleander (*Nerium oleander* L. [synonym *Nerium indicum* Mill.])
  Periwinkle (*Catharanthus roseus* [L.] G. Don)
  Plumeria (*Plumeria* species)

**Heath Family, Ericaceae**
  Azalea (*Rhododendron* species)

**Lily Family, Liliaceae**
  Gloriosa Lily (*Gloriosa superba* L.)

**Mahogany Family, Meliaceae**
  Chinaberry (*Melia azedarach* L.)

**Mango Family, Anacardiaceae**
  Cashew (*Anacardium occidentale* L.)
  Mango (*Mangifera indica* L.)

**Milkweed Family, Asclepiadaceae**
  Crown Flower (*Calotropis gigantea* [L.] W. T. Aiton)

## Nightshade Family, Solanaceae

Angel's Trumpet (*Brugmansia* × *candida* Pers.
[also called *Datura candida*])
Cestrum (*Cestrum* species)
Cup of Gold and Silver Cup (*Solandra* species)
Jimsonweed (*Datura stramonium* L.)
Nightshade (*Solanum* species)

## Pea Family, Fabaceae

Black-Eyed Susan (*Abrus precatorius* L.)

## Pepper Family, Piperaceae

Kava (*Piper methysticum* G. Forster)

## Philodendron Family, Araceae

Anthurium (*Anthurium* species)
Dumb Cane (*Dieffenbachia* species)
Elephant Ear (*Alocasia* and *Xanthosoma* species)
Taro (*Colocasia esculenta* [L.] Schott)

## Pokeweed Family, Phytolacca

Pokeberry (*Phytolacca* species)
Coral Berry (*Rivina humilis* L.)

## Poppy Family, Papaveraceae

Hawaiian Poppy (*Argemone glauca* [Prain] Pope)

## Protea Family, Proteaceae

*Kāhili* Flower (*Grevillea banksii* R. Br.)
Silky Oak (*Grevillea robusta* R. Br.)

## Saxifrage Family, Saxifragaceae

Hydrangea (*Hydrangea macrophylla* [Thunb.] Ser.)

## Snapdragon Family, Scrophulariaceae

Foxglove (*Digitalis purpurea* L.)

## Spurge Family, Euphorbiaceae

Cassava (*Manihot esculenta* Crantz)
Castor Bean (*Ricinus communis* L.)
Candlenut (*Aleurites moluccana* [L.] Willd.)
Crown of Thorns (*Euphorbia milli* Des Moul.)
Jatropha (*Jatropha* species)
Pencil Plant (*Euphorbia tirucalli* L.)
Poinsettia (*Euphorbia pulcherrima* Klotzsch)
Red Spurge (*Euphorbia cotinifolia* L.)
Slipper Flower (*Pedilanthus tithymaloides* [L.] Poito.)

## Verbena Family, Verbenaceae

Lantana (*Lantana camara* L.)

## Mushroom Order, Agaricales, Includes Thirteen Families Found in Hawai'i

Tricholomataceae, 99 species
Coprinaceae, 30 species
Agaricaceae, 28 species
Entolomataceae, 19 species
Cortinariaceae, 17 species
Hygrophoraceae, 12 species
Crepidotaceae, 12 species
Strophariaceae, 11 species
Bolbitiaceae, 9 species
Pluteaceae, 9 species
Boletaceae, 5 species
Amanitaceae, 2 species
Paxillaceae, 2 species

# Quick Guide to Poisonous Plants in Hawai'i

| PLANT | FREQUENCY OF POISONING | MEDICALLY DANGEROUS? | CLASSIC SYMPTOMS |
|---|---|---|---|
| **Allamanda** *Allamanda cathartica* | Rare | No | Vomiting, diarrhea |
| **Angel's trumpet** *Brugmansia x candida* | Occasional | Yes | Dilated pupils, dry mouth, red skin, delirium |
| **Anthurium** *Anthurium* species | Common | No | Pain and swelling of lips, mouth, tongue, and throat |
| **Azalea** *Rhododendron* species | Rare | Yes | Mouth tingling, vomiting, sweating, slow heart rate |
| **Be-still tree** *Thevetia peruviana* | Rare | Yes | Irregular heartbeat, confusion, headaches |
| **Black-eyed Susan** *Abrus precatorius* | Rare | Yes | Bloody vomiting and bloody diarrhea |
| **Candlenut** *Aleurites moluccana* | Common | No | Vomiting, diarrhea |
| **Cashew-nut tree** *Anacardium occidentale* | Rare | No | Rash from handling raw nuts |
| **Cassava** *Manihot esculenta* | Rare | Yes | Dizziness, fatigue, rapid breathing |
| **Castor bean** *Ricinus communis* | Rare | Yes | Bloody vomiting and bloody diarrhea |
| **Cerbera** *Cerbera manghas* | Rare | Yes | Irregular heartbeat, confusion, headaches |
| **Cestrum** *Cestrum* species | Rare | Yes | Extremely variable |
| **Chinaberry** *Melia azedarach* | Rare | Yes | Dilated pupils, teeth grinding, paralysis |
| **Crown flower** *Calotropis gigantea* | Rare | Yes | Irregular heartbeat, confusion, headaches |
| **Cup of gold and silver cup** *Solandra* species | Rare | Yes | Extremely variable |
| **Dumb cane** *Dieffenbachia* species | Common | Yes | Pain and swelling of lips, mouth, tongue, and throat |
| **Elephant ear** *Alocasia* species and *Xanthosoma* species | Common | Occasionally | Pain and swelling of lips, mouth, tongue, and throat |
| **Foxglove** *Digitalis purpurea* | Rare | Yes | Irregular heartbeat, confusion, headaches |
| **Gloriosa lily** | R | Y | Numb mouth, chest pain, rapid heartbeat |

| PLANT | FREQUENCY OF POISONING | MEDICALLY DANGEROUS? | CLASSIC SYMPTOMS |
|---|---|---|---|
| **Hawaiian poppy**<br>*Argemone glauca* | Rare | Unknown | Visual disturbance, abdominal swelling, fainting |
| **Hydrangea**<br>*Hydrangea macrophylla* | Occasional | Yes | Dizziness, fatigue, rapid breathing |
| **Japanese anemone**<br>*Anemone hupehensis* | Rare | Occasionally | Mouth burning, blisters |
| **Jatropha plants**<br>*Jatropha* species | Rare | Yes | Bloody vomiting, bloody diarrhea |
| **Jimsonweed**<br>*Datura stramonium* | Occasional | Yes | Dilated pupils, dry mouth, red skin, delirium |
| **Kāhili flower and silky oak**<br>*Grevillea* species | Rare | No | Rash from handling |
| **Kava**<br>*Piper methysticum* | Occasional | No | Sedation, scaly rash, stomach pain |
| **Lantana**<br>*Lantana camara* | Rare | Occasionally | Dilated pupils, delirium |
| **Mango**<br>*Mangifera indica* | Common | No | Rash from handling |
| **Mushrooms**<br>Agaricales | Occasional | Occasionally | Vomiting, diarrhea |
| **Nightshade**<br>*Solanum* species | Rare | Yes | Extremely variable |
| **Oleander**<br>*Nerium oleander* | Rare | Yes | Irregular heartbeat, confusion, headache |
| **Pencil plant, crown-of-thorns, red spurge, and slipper flower**<br>*Euphorbia* and *Pedilanthus* species | Occasional | No | Rash, mouth burning, stomach pain |
| **Periwinkle**<br>*Catharanthus roseus* | Rare | Yes | Numbness, tingling, and weakness |
| **Plumeria**<br>*Plumeria* species | Common | No | Rash, diarrhea |
| **Poinsettia**<br>*Euphorbia pulcherrima* | Common | No | Mouth irritation |
| **Pokeberry and coral berry**<br>*Phytolacca* species and *Rivina humilis* | Rare | Occasionally | Mouth burning, bloody foamy diarrhea |
| **Star-of-Bethlehem**<br>*Hippobroma longiflora* | Rare | Yes | Metallic taste, profuse salivation |
| **Taro**<br>*Colocasia esculenta* | Common | No | Pain and swelling of lips, mouth, tongue, and throat |

# ALLAMANDA
## *(Allamanda cathartica)*

Allamanda is a sprawling vine native to Brazil. People grow these vines in parks, gardens, and yards for the fragrant, yellow flowers, about 3 inches wide. Because the vines rarely bear fruit in Hawai'i, new plants are made from cuttings.

Species of allamanda other than *Allamanda cathartica* have smaller, pink flowers and bear fruit. These species are less common in Hawai'i than the yellow ones.

Allamanda vines are popular ornamental flowers, common throughout Hawai'i, Florida, and the Caribbean Islands, where they adorn homes, fences, and trellises. The Hawaiian name, *nani ali'i* (also *lani ali'i*), means chiefly beauty.

## Toxin

The toxin in allamanda is an unknown cathartic. All parts of the plant are mildly toxic to suck on or eat.

The white, milky fluid in the leaves, stems, and flowers may irritate skin and eyes.

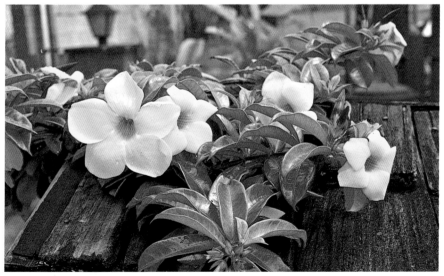

Yellow allamanda is a common flowering vine in Hawai'i. All of the plant is mildly toxic to suck on or eat but is not medically dangerous. Some people develop a rash after handling allamanda. *(Susan Scott)*

# Traditional and Modern Uses

In India, some people consider 1 to 2 grains (0.003 to 0.006 oz.) of allamanda bark an excellent laxative.

People in Columbia once drank the white sap of allamanda as a treatment for worms, but no one knows if or how this treatment affected the worms. The practice was abandoned because it often caused vomiting and diarrhea.

Cubans still occasionally drink allamanda sap, or a tea made from the leaves, as a drastic laxative treatment and to induce vomiting.

Using allamanda as a remedy is scientifically unproven and may be harmful.

# Incidence

Allamandas are common in Hawai'i, but they are not a common cause of illness or skin rash in the Islands. In 1997 and 1998, the Hawai'i Poison Center received no calls about allamanda exposure.

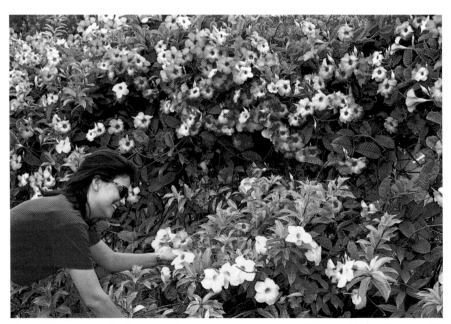

The pink species of allamanda is less common in Hawai'i than the yellow. Both species carry the same mild toxin. *(Susan Scott)*

# Signs and Symptoms

Children have been known to lick these flowers, but they usually do not swallow enough of the toxin to become ill.

In one case, a six-year-old boy who sucked on allamanda stems became nauseated. The next day, he developed a fever, swollen lips, dry mouth, and thirst.

Another child, after picking allamanda flowers, wiped her sticky fingers on the bare skin of her side. The skin developed an itchy rash the next day.

A woman who got allamanda sap in her eye reported a strong burning sensation.

In small doses, allamanda leaves, stems, and flowers produce diarrhea. Larger amounts cause violent vomiting and diarrhea. Regularly drinking allamanda tea causes chronic diarrhea.

 ## First Aid

Usually, the nausea, vomiting, diarrhea, and/or rash produced by this plant disappear without treatment.

If allamanda sap gets in the eyes, rinse with large amounts of tap water. See a physician for persistent burning or if blurred vision develops.

For rash, wash the area thoroughly with soap and water. If itching persists, try 1 percent hydrocortisone cream 4 times a day, and 1 or 2 25-milligram diphenhydramine (Benadryl) tablets every 6 hours. Diphenhydramine may cause drowsiness: Do not drive, swim, or surf after taking this medication. Give itching children diphenhydramine syrup, following the dosage directions on the package.

For hives or persistent vomiting and diarrhea, go to an emergency room. For facial swelling, any difficulty breathing, or collapse, call 911. Take flowers, stems, and leaves of the plant to the emergency room for identification.

 ## Advanced Medical Treatment

No specific antidote or clinically useful diagnostic test exists for allamanda rash or poisoning. Most cases are mild and respond to first aid.

Decontaminate skin and/or eyes. There are no reports of serious corneal injury.

Give charcoal for ingestions; replace fluids and electrolytes as needed.

# ANGEL'S TRUMPET
## (*Brugmansia* x *candida*)

Hawai'i's angel's trumpet tree (also known as *Datura candida*) is a hybrid of two species of angel's trumpets native to the Andes.

The first angel's trumpet tree in Hawai'i came from Rio de Janeiro on the frigate *Blonde* in 1825. Today, these lovely plants grow throughout Hawai'i as sweet-smelling ornamental shrubs or trees.

The Hawaiian name for the flowers, *nānāhonua*, means gazing earthward, referring to the 10-inch-long, trumpet-

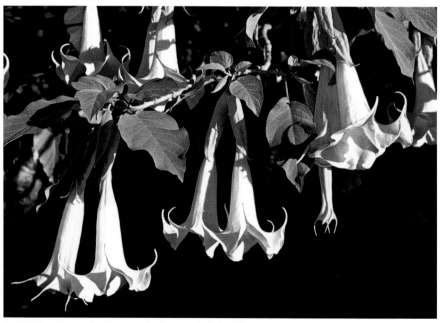

All parts of angel's trumpet plants contain alkaloids that can cause hallucinations if eaten or drunk as tea. The hallucinations are usually terrifying, and other effects of the plant are unpleasant. (*Susan Scott*)

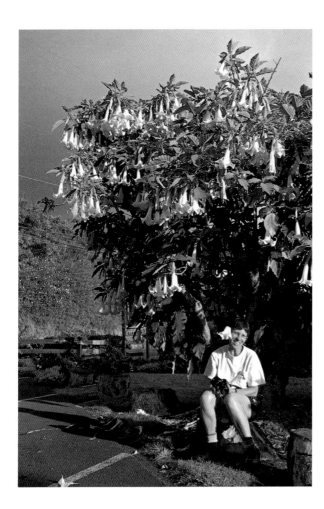

Angel's trumpet trees can grow to about 12 feet tall. The scent of the flowers is pleasant but can make some people feel ill. Tucking one of the flowers behind the ear, as the author did in this photo, has also made people ill (though it did not in this case). Presumably, the skin behind the ear can absorb the flower's toxins. *(Craig Thomas)*

shaped flowers that hang from the tree. The flowers are white or pale pink; their fragrance is strongest at night.

In Hawai'i, people sometimes call angel's trumpets belladonna, though belladonna *(Atropa belladonna)* is a different plant and is not found in the Islands. The word *belladonna* means beautiful lady in Italian. (This name was given to the *Atropa* plant in the fourteenth century because eating some of the plant or rubbing it in the eyes caused women's pupils to dilate. Apparently, large, dark pupils were regarded as a beautiful feature.)

The toxins of angel's trumpets and belladonna are closely related.

# Toxin

The entire angel's trumpet plant is toxic, containing the alkaloids atropine, hyoscyamine, and scopolamine. Scopolamine, the principal active compound in angel's trumpets, affects the central nervous system.

# Traditional and Modern Uses

Angel's trumpets are closely related to jimsonweed and other members of the *Datura* genus. American Indians, people practicing traditional Chinese medicine, and modern pharmaceutical companies have long used these plants as medicines. One common practice in several areas of the world has been to inhale smoke from the burning leaves of this plant to relieve asthma. This and other traditional uses of the plant are scientifically unproven and may be harmful. (See Jimsonweed for more detailed uses of this group of plants.)

Though angel's trumpets are grown almost exclusively as ornamental trees in Hawai'i, some people believe they can get a drug-induced high, or hallucinate, from eating the flowers or leaves. While it is true the drugs in this plant can cause hallucinations, they are often terrifying, and other effects of the drugs are unpleasant.

# Incidence

In 1997, the Hawaii Poison Center received calls from three people with angel's trumpet exposures; in 1998, three victims called.

One 1995 Hawai'i report tells of a nineteen-year-old military man who drank tea made from steeping angel's trumpet flowers. He cried, became confused, felt happiness, then anger, then sadness. When the symptoms continued the next morning, his friends took him to an emergency room. He recovered in twenty-four hours except for blurred vision, which took several days to disappear.

Children can accidentally be poisoned if they put these flowers in their mouths or even if they pretend to blow them like trumpets. A Florida boy appeared deeply drugged after falling asleep in a hammock under a blooming angel's trumpet tree. He recovered. Some native Colombians believe that sleeping under a blooming angel's trumpet tree can be fatal.

In Canada, in the 1980s, two people were poisoned after eating hamburgers accidentally seasoned with seeds from angel's trumpets. They lost consciousness, but recovered in twenty-four hours.

Several people in Hong Kong became ill after taking the traditional Chinese medicine *ling-xiao-hua*. Researchers later determined that the medicine mistakenly contained *Datura metel* flowers, a close relative of angel's trumpets.

## Signs and Symptoms

Most people enjoy the scent of angel's trumpets, but some people suffer headache, nausea, dizziness, and weakness after smelling them when the flowers are in full bloom.

Rubbing one or both eyes after handling this plant may cause the pupil(s) to dilate. This causes blurred vision and sensitivity to bright light, which can last for about a week.

Symptoms of angel's trumpet poisoning usually occur within 30 to 60 minutes after eating and may last for 24 to 48 hours.

Initial symptoms of mild to moderate poisoning after eating or drinking tea made from angel's trumpet include warm skin, dilated pupils (causing blurred vision and sensitivity to bright light), dry mouth (causing difficulty swallowing and speaking), reddening of the face, restlessness, irritability, disorientation, hallucinations, and/or delirium. Blurred vision and dilated pupils from eating angel's trumpet plants may last 7 to 12 days.

In severe poisonings, victims may feel cold, may become agitated and combative, may be unable to urinate, may have seizures, paralysis, coma, respiratory failure, circulation collapse, and may die.

To remember the varied signs and symptoms of this class of drug intoxication, medical doctors traditionally memorize the following phrase: "Hot as a hare, blind as a bat, dry as a bone, red as a beet, and mad as a hatter."

 ## First Aid

Wash hands thoroughly after handling angel's trumpet flowers or leaves. Rinse exposed eyes with copious amounts of tap water. For persistent blurred vision, consult a doctor.

Mild to moderate cases of angel's trumpet poisoning usually disappear overnight without treatment. If symptoms are severe, take the victim to an emergency room. For facial swelling, any difficulty breathing, or collapse, call 911. Take flowers, stems, and leaves of the plant to the emergency room for identification.

## Advanced Medical Treatment

No specific antidote or clinically useful diagnostic test exists for angel's trumpet poisoning, which presents as atropine poisoning. Make the diagnosis by physical exam and history.

Scopolamine and atropine impair peristalsis. Therefore, in severe poisonings, consider emptying the stomach even if more than an hour has elapsed since ingestion. For all ingestions, give charcoal. Catheterize for urinary retention. Use diazepam as necessary for sedation.

Consider physostigmine only for uncontrollable hyperthermia, supraventricular tachycardia with hemodynamic instability, therapy-resistant seizures, and extreme delirium. The recommended dose of physostigmine in adults is 1 to 2 milligrams intravenously over 5 minutes. Repeat every 15 minutes as needed. Never exceed 4 mg in 30 minutes.[1]

For children, start with 0.02 milligrams per kilogram, increasing dose as necessary to 0.5 mg. Repeat as needed to control symptoms. The maximum dose is 2 mg.[2]

Physostigmine dramatically reverses coma and other anticholinergic symptoms but may itself cause seizures. Never use physostigmine just to keep a patient awake.

# ANTHURIUM
## (*Anthurium* species)

Anthuriums are native to tropical America; more than seven hundred species exist in the world. Many of these, and some hybrids, are grown commercially in Hawai'i as potted plants, garden plants, or for cut flowers. These heart-shaped, showy flowers bear a long spike at the base. Bright red anthuriums are common in gardens and bouquets throughout Hawai'i.

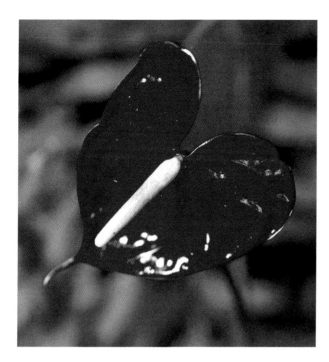

There are more than 700 kinds of anthuriums in the world. In Hawai'i, these red ones are common in bouquets and gardens. Anthuriums are not dangerously poisonous. (Susan Scott)

# Toxin

All parts of the anthurium plant may contain bundles of needlelike calcium oxalate crystals, but most are in the leaves and stems. Calcium oxalate is a nonabsorbable salt of oxalic acid, a colorless, crystalline, potentially poisonous organic acid found in many common food plants, such as spinach, rhubarb, tomatoes, grapes, and sweet potatoes. The human body produces its own oxalic acid. Some kidney stones contain calcium oxalate.

Whether eating calcium oxalate crystals is harmful depends on the cooking methods and on its concentration in a particular plant. Some plants bearing this substance require no cooking, others require considerable cooking, and some cannot be made edible by any amount of cooking.

The amount of calcium oxalate in a plant varies greatly from species to species and often even within the same species. The toxicity of anthurium plants is questionable among researchers; some do not list anthuriums as toxic; others do.

Juices from these plants may cause a skin rash.

No one uses anthuriums for food, but the eye-catching spike

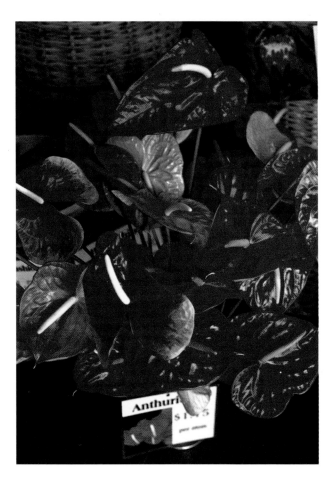

Vases containing bright red anthuriums can be tempting to young children, who sometimes put the flowers into their mouths. Unless the child actually chews the flowers, this usually causes little or no harm. *(Susan Scott)*

and red color attract toddlers, who often grab a flower and stuff it into their mouths. A child, however, would have to crush or chew the leaf, flower, or stem to produce symptoms. Mechanical action like this causes special cells in the plant to inject the needle-sharp calcium oxalate crystals into the skin or mucosa. Chewing also causes the release of an enzyme that produces redness and swelling.

Brief sucking on, or licking of, a leaf or flower is not usually toxic.

## Traditional and Modern Uses

In Hawai'i and throughout the world, anthuriums are common flowers in tropical bouquets and in gardens.

# Incidence

In 1997, the Hawaii Poison Center received a call from one person whose child had eaten an anthurium; in 1998, eight people called. These numbers represent only a small fraction of the number of anthurium exposures experienced by Hawai'i residents and visitors. Because anthuriums are so plentiful in Hawai'i, incidents of children putting these flowers into their mouths are fairly common. Usually, symptoms are nonexistent or mild.

# Signs and Symptoms

Anthurium sap or juice on the skin may cause a red, itching rash. Sap in the eyes may cause immediate pain, tearing, and sensitivity to light.

The main symptom of eating calcium oxalate crystals is immediate pain followed by swelling of the lips, mouth, tongue, and throat. Some describe it as pins-and-needles pain. The victim often has excessive salivation, and blisters sometimes develop. Speaking may be difficult or impossible for up to 2 days. Swelling of the throat may make breathing difficult.

If a child swallows any of the plant, vomiting and diarrhea may follow.

 # First Aid

The pain and swelling on the skin and in the mouth from calcium oxalate crystals usually disappear slowly without special therapy.

Wash exposed skin thoroughly with soap and water. Try removing embedded crystals with sticky tape. If the rash itches persistently, try 1 percent hydrocortisone cream 4 times a day, and 1 or 2 25-milligram diphenhydramine (Benadryl) tablets every 6 hours. Diphenhydramine may cause drowsiness: Do not drive, swim, or surf after taking this medication. Give children diphenhydramine syrup, following the dosage directions on the package.

For plant juice in the eyes, rinse with large amounts of tap water for at least 15 minutes. Go to an emergency room for blurry vision, swelling, or prolonged pain.

For anthurium plants in the mouth, remove the plant part immediately and rinse the mouth with large amounts of water, instructing the child to spit out the water. Later, sucking on ice cubes may help relieve pain. Have the child spit out, not swallow, the ice water.

If swelling occurs in the face, mouth, or throat, or if the victim has any difficulty breathing, call 911 for help. Take the whole plant to the emergency room for identification.

## Advanced Medical Treatment

No specific antidote or clinically useful diagnostic test exists for calcium oxalate rash, eye exposure, or ingestion. Most cases have only local symptoms, which usually respond to first aid treatment.

Calcium oxalate crystals do not dissolve in the digestive tract and therefore do not cause systemic poisoning. They can, however, cause severe, burning pain, hematemesis, and bloody diarrhea.

Sap in the eyes may cause corneal abrasions or deposits of calcium oxalate crystals on the cornea. Irrigate thoroughly and examine with a slit lamp. Ocular steroids are unproven but may decrease pain.

Pain medication may be necessary for both ocular and oral pain.

# AZALEA
## (*Rhododendron* species)

About 850 species of rhododendrons exist in the world. These 5 to 6 feet–tall shrubs are cultivated worldwide for their stunning, rounded clusters of white, pink, red, purple, yellow, or orange flowers. Most rhododendrons come from temperate regions of the Northern Hemisphere.

Azaleas are a type of rhododendron. Hawai'i's azaleas, mainly *Rhododendron simsii* and *R. macrosepalum*, and their hybrids, are native to Asia. People often grow these flowering azaleas in pots on the *lānai* or in gardens. They are also common bushes in parks, blooming profusely from late fall through spring.

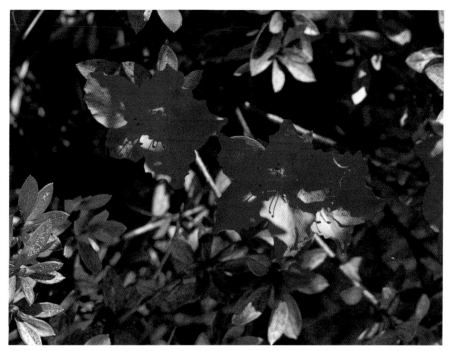

Azaleas, common as shrubs and potted plants in Hawai'i, are a type of rhododendron. All parts of all rhododendrons are moderately poisonous to eat but safe to handle. *(Susan Scott)*

# Toxin

The entire rhododendron plant—flowers, leaves, and stems—may be moderately poisonous to eat, particularly the leaves.

The toxins in rhododendrons are grayanotoxins, resinoid substances that bind to sodium channels in cell membranes, thus keeping the channels open. This interferes with the function of the heart, skeletal muscles, and central nervous system.

Frequent crossing of species and hybridization of azaleas and other rhododendrons result in wide variability in the potency of the poisons from one plant to another. Though the toxicity of azaleas is unpredictable, eating less than about three azalea leaves or flowers should not cause symptoms. Conversely, eating only one teaspoon of honey containing azalea nectar has made people sick. This is sometimes called mad honey poisoning.

Handling the flowers and stems in bouquets is safe.

## Traditional and Modern Uses

People have been known to smoke rhododendron plant parts for unknown medicinal purposes and become ill from it. Using any part of a rhododendron plant as a remedy is scientifically unproven and dangerous; it may cause death.

## Incidence

Azaleas are not a common cause of poisoning in Hawai'i. In 1997, the Hawaii Poison Center received only one call from a person exposed to azaleas; in 1998, there were no calls.

In other parts of the world, children have been poisoned by sucking nectar from azalea and other rhododendron flowers. Honey contaminated with rhododendron nectar has also poisoned people.

In the distant past, people occasionally died from rhododendron poisoning, but no deaths have been reported in modern times.

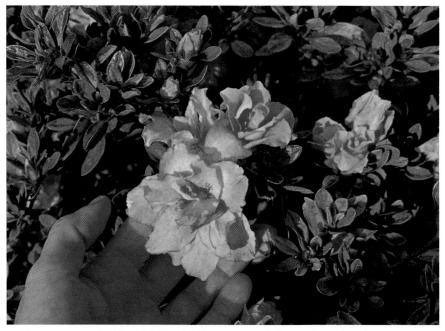

With so many azalea hybrids, their degree of toxicity varies. It is safest to regard all azaleas as poisonous. *(Susan Scott)*

# Signs and Symptoms

Symptoms do not always occur, but if they do, the first effects are burning, numbness, and tingling of the mouth. Often, nausea follows, with vomiting, excessive sweating, general muscle weakness, low blood pressure, and slow (or sometimes fast) heartbeat. Occasionally, a victim will experience temporary blindness or blurred vision.

Extreme poisoning can progress to confusion, seizures, and coma. Symptoms begin from 30 minutes to 2 hours after eating contaminated honey. Rhododendron poisoning symptoms do not usually last more than 24 hours.

 ## First Aid

If you see a child eating the flowers or leaves of an azalea, or if a person becomes ill after eating honey, take them to an emergency room. For facial swelling, any difficulty breathing, or collapse, call 911. Take flowers, stems, and leaves of the plant to the emergency room for identification.

 ## Advanced Medical Treatment

No diagnostic or clinically useful test exists for grayanotoxins.

Direct treatment at controlling emesis. Give charcoal; replace fluids and electrolytes as needed. Other treatment for severe rhododendron poisoning is supportive. Be prepared to treat hypotension, bradycardia, and seizures. Rarely, patients experience altered levels of consciousness; be prepared to protect the airway.

The prognosis of rhododendron poisoning is excellent.

# BE-STILL TREE
## (Thevetia peruviana)

*Thevetia peruviana* is a small tree native to tropical America. In Hawaiian, it is known as *nohomālie*. People transported be-still trees to Hawai'i around 1900 to grow as ornamental shrubs. Today, these trees are common in gardens and parks throughout the Islands; occasionally, they grow wild. Their yellow, trumpet-shaped flowers bloom year round. Be-still trees bearing pinkish flowers are also present in Hawai'i but are less common than the yellow variety.

The long, narrow leaves of these trees make them easy to identify. The fruits usually bear two to four shiny, flat, black seeds, called lucky nuts among some Caribbean Islanders.

Be-still trees are often referred to as yellow oleander. Though be-still trees are not close relatives of oleander bushes, both contain potentially lethal heart toxins. Be-still trees also contain a white sap that can cause rashes.

## Toxins

All parts of the be-still tree contain the cardiac glycosides peruvoside and thevetin A and B. Cardiac glycosides block normal electrical impulses throughout the body, including the heart, by

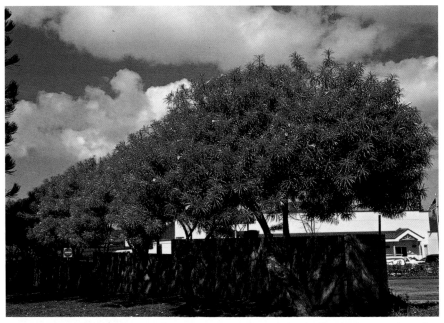

Because be-still trees bear yellow flowers and contain similar toxins as oleander shrubs, they are often called yellow oleander. Despite their potentially deadly toxins, and the common occurrence of these small trees in parks and gardens throughout Hawai'i, poisonings from them are rare. *(Susan Scott)*

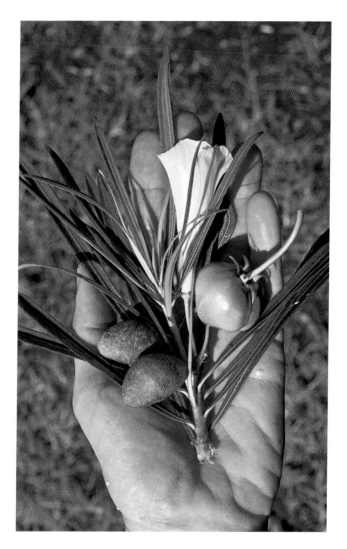

All parts of be-still trees contain a dangerous heart toxin. Never use the wood as fuel or sticks from this tree as skewers to cook food. Be-still seeds have a particularly high concentration of toxin. *(Susan Scott)*

interfering with the exchange of sodium and potassium in and out of nerve and muscle cells.

Though cardiac glycosides are found throughout the tree, the seeds have the highest concentration. One seed can kill a child; eight to ten can kill an adult.

People experience a wide range of responses after eating plants containing cardiac glycosides. Some barely become sick; others have died. Regard all parts of this plant as extremely toxic, whether the parts are green, dry, or burning. Never use a stick from a be-still tree to roast marshmallows or hot dogs.

An unknown toxin in be-still trees causes kidney and liver damage when eaten. Be-still trees also contain gums and oils that can cause a blistering rash on the skin and irritate the eyes.

Inhaling plant dust while raking be-still leaves may irritate the nose and throat. Inhaling smoke from burning be-still trees can cause poisoning.

## Traditional and Modern Uses

People in some areas of the world use parts of be-still trees to kill insects, fish, and other animals. Others use the sap, bark, leaves, and seeds as folk medicine. Such traditional uses of this plant are scientifically unproven, extremely dangerous, and may cause serious illness or death.

In the Caribbean Islands, people carry or wear polished be-still seeds as good luck charms. Some believe carrying these seeds will prevent the occurrence of hemorrhoids.

Researchers used be-still seed extracts in the 1930s to treat people with heart failure and atrial fibrillation. Hundreds of pounds of be-still seeds were once shipped from Honolulu for such pharmaceutical use. Today, drug companies make similar heart medicines synthetically.

## Incidence

Poisonings from be-still trees are rare, probably because the seeds are bitter tasting and produce nearly instant vomiting. In 1997, the Hawaii Poison Center received calls from two people exposed to be-still trees; in 1998, there were no calls.

Though poisonings from these trees are rare, at least two deaths have been reported in Hawai‘i. Both were children who ate an unknown number of seeds. Deaths have also been reported in Florida, Australia, and South Africa.

Most poisoning cases are in children who accidentally eat seeds while playing near be-still trees; most adult cases are suicides or homicides. The use of be-still tree ingredients in folk medicine has caused serious illness and death.

Poisoning may also occur if a person inhales smoke from a fire made from the wood and branches of be-still trees, or roasts hot dogs or marshmallows on sticks cut from the tree.

# Signs and Symptoms

Be-still sap in the eyes causes redness, pain, and tearing. The pupils may dilate, causing blurred vision. Sap on the skin may cause red, painful bumps or blisters.

People who eat any part of a be-still tree, especially the seeds, may have immediate burning, redness, and swelling of the lips and mouth. Swallowing this plant can cause the victim to have nausea, vomiting, abdominal pain, and cramping. This can go on for several hours before generalized heart symptoms begin, which include slow or irregular heartbeat, dizziness, headache, and confusion. Victims may feel drowsy or giddy.

Death has occurred from 2 to 24 hours after eating be-still seeds.

## First Aid

Thoroughly wash skin exposed to the sap of this tree with soap and water. For persistent redness, swelling, or pain in the area, consult a doctor.

Rinse exposed eyes for at least 15 minutes with tap water. For persistent itching or blurred vision, consult a doctor.

Regard as a medical emergency the swallowing of any part of this plant or the inhaling of smoke from it. Call 911. Take seeds, flowers, and a branch from the tree to the emergency room for identification.

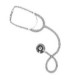

## Advanced Medical Treatment

No specific treatment exists for eye irritation or dermatitis from be-still tree sap. Use standard therapy to treat symptoms.

In be-still tree poisonings, hypertension is common in early stages; hypotension develops later.

The effects of the cardiac glycocides peruvoside and thevetin A and B are similar to digoxin and digitoxin. Therefore, laboratory tests for these drugs may be positive for some (but not all) be-still poisonings. Because these tests rely on cross-reactivity between the plant's cardiac glycosides and digoxin or digitoxin, serum levels do not necessarily correlate with biological activity. A low digoxin or digitoxin level may indicate a potentially fatal level of be-still cardiac glycosides.

An elevated potassium level in the presence of a plant ingestion suggests cardiac glycoside exposure.

If the patient has swallowed be-still an hour or less before going to the ER, empty the stomach. For all patients suspected of eating any part of a be-still tree, regardless of time elapsed, give charcoal.

Victims suspected of eating plants containing cardiac glycosides require cardiac monitoring. However, the effect of cardiac glycosides on the heart may be delayed; monitor asymptomatic patients for at least 12 hours before discharge.

For life-threatening arrythmias, hyperkalemia, prolonged PR intervals, widened QRS segments, or altered mental status, administer 10 vials of digoxin immune FAB intravenously. In one case of cardiac glycoside poisoning from oleander, the patient woke up 4 minutes after FAB treatment was begun, and his potassium level normalized in 1 hour. If improvement is minimal, give another 10 vials. The cross-reactivity for binding may require a high concentration of digoxin immune FAB.

The risks of digoxin immune FAB include fever, apnea, hypokalemia, and hypoglycemia. Rebound toxicity occurs in 3 to 11 days in a small fraction of patients treated with digoxin immune FAB. Some researchers suggest a continuous FAB infusion after an initial bolus. Hemoperfusion and forced diuresis are of no benefit.

If FAB is unavailable, use IV atropine to treat bradycardia, and lidocaine, amiodarone, or phenytoin for ventricular arrythmias. Consider phenytoin or a pacemaker in victims with second- or third-degree heart block.

A study of ten patients who survived be-still seed poisoning revealed that all of them developed hemolytic jaundice, hemoglobinuria, and fever the second day after the poisoning. These conditions resolved without specific treatment.

# BLACK-EYED SUSAN
## (Abrus precatorius)

*Abrus precatorius* is a vine that climbs over other plants and to the tops of small trees. The vine's flowers and seed pods resemble those of peas. Native to Africa and tropical Asia,

*Abrus precatorius* has been in Hawai'i at least since 1871. It is a common plant in tropical areas throughout the world.

In Hawai'i and Florida, people often refer to *Abrus precatorius* as black-eyed Susan, but it is not related to the yellow garden flower commonly known as black-eyed Susan nor is it related to the twining plant known as the black-eyed Susan vine *(Thunbergia allata)*.

*Abrus precatorius* has many other common names, including jequirity bean, rosary pea, coral pea, crab's eyes, bead vine, and precatory bean.

People in Hawai'i cultivate *Abrus precatorius* for its beautiful red seeds, each bearing a black "eye." The plants also grow wild at low elevations in dry, disturbed areas, particularly in the Kona and Puna districts on the island of Hawai'i.

When the green pods of these plants ripen, they turn brown, then curl open to drop their four to eight seeds. These seeds can be deadly.

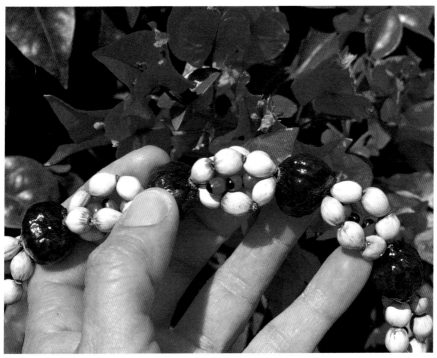

These black-tipped, red seeds are called black-eyed Susans in Hawai'i, where they are sometimes used in necklaces, like this one, bought near Kalapana on the Island of Hawai'i. The red seeds are extremely toxic. *(Susan Scott)*

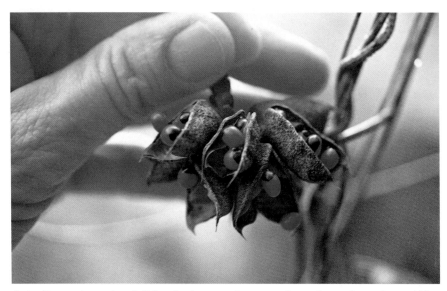

Only the red seeds of this plant are poisonous. One chewed seed can kill a person, and a needle-prick while stringing the seeds in *lei* can cause serious illness. *(Susan Scott)*

## Toxin

Black-eyed Susan seeds contain a potentially lethal toxin called abrin, a type of toxalbumin. The rest of the plant is not toxic.

Toxalbumins cause severe, bleeding lesions in the mouth, esophagus, stomach, and intestines. The lesions are similar to alkaline burns, though the onset is delayed several hours after ingestion. Once absorbed into the bloodstream, toxalbumins interfere with cell function and cause cell damage, leading to serious liver, kidney, adrenal, and nerve damage.

Toxalbumins are so potent that one raw, chewed seed can kill a human.

Though not closely related scientifically to the black-eyed Susan, castor beans and *Jatropha* species also contain toxalbumins.

## Traditional and Modern Uses

Black-eyed Susan seeds are so reliably uniform in weight and size that people in India use them in balances to weigh jewels and precious metals. Throughout the world, people use these lovely seeds in jewelry, rosaries, and home decorations. In Hawai'i, *lei* makers string the red seeds into *lei*, and jewelry makers use them in necklaces.

In Africa and Madagascar, people once used black-eyed Susan seeds as ordeal poison: If the accused survived the ordeal of eating some of the seeds, they were judged innocent of the offense in question; if they died, they were presumed to have been guilty. Africans also once (but not presently) used black-eyed Susan infusions in the eyes to treat various eye maladies. Abortionists have used black-eyed Susan seeds to induce abortions. The use of black-eyed Susan seeds as a remedy for anything is extremely dangerous and may cause death.

In India, criminals have ground these seeds into a paste, then fashioned the paste into tiny, pointed cylinders. A potential murderer then inserted the cylinder beneath the skin of his or her victim. Death occurred in a few hours.

## Incidence

In 1997, the Hawaii Poison Center received one call from a person exposed to a black-eyed Susan seed; in 1998, one person called. The outcome of these incidents is unknown.

In other parts of the world, children have died from eating only one immature black-eyed Susan seed.

Because black-eyed Susan seed coats are hard, people can survive unharmed if they swallow intact seeds whole. Thus, the degree of poisoning a person experiences depends on how thoroughly the victim chewed the seeds.

People have also been poisoned when the toxin was absorbed through a cut or open sore. A needle prick while stringing seeds has caused serious poisoning.

These seeds are supposedly harmless if cooked for several hours; people in Micronesia reportedly eat them like cooked beans. However, given their potential deadliness, it is wise to avoid eating these seeds under any circumstances.

## Signs and Symptoms

Pricking a finger while stringing black-eyed Susan seeds can cause immediate painful swelling, a cold sweat, and throat and nasal congestion.

In the eyes, juice from these seeds can cause redness, tearing and swelling, and destruction of eye tissue, depending on the concentration.

After swallowing broken or chewed black-eyed Susan seeds, symptoms do not usually begin for 6 hours to 3 days. Then, the victim has a burning sensation in the mouth and throat, followed by nausea, vomiting, and diarrhea, often with bleeding. In severe cases, open sores form in the mouth, esophagus, and throughout the stomach and intestines. These symptoms look like chemical burns. Blood in the urine is common.

Dehydration follows. Death occurs as a result of fluid loss.

## First Aid

Getting black-eyed Susan seed toxin under the skin by a needle prick, in the eyes, or in the body by swallowing is always a medical emergency. Call 911. Take the seeds, and the rest of the plant if available, to the emergency room for identification.

## Advanced Medical Treatment

No specific antidote or clinically useful diagnostic test exists for toxalbumin poisoning. Make the diagnosis by physical exam and history.

Either absorbed through a cut or eaten, this toxin is life-threatening because of potential shock from fluid and electrolyte loss. Decontaminate exposed skin and eyes. Examine eyes with a slit lamp and perform funduscopic exam to check for both pupillary dilation and constriction. Retinal hemorrhage and optic neuritis have been reported.

Gastrointestinal injury is similar to caustic alkaline burns, though the onset is delayed 2 to 3 hours after ingestion.

Keep asymptomatic patients suspected of swallowing one or more seeds under observation for at least 8 hours. Instruct care-givers to call 911 immediately if symptoms begin later at home.

For ingestions, give charcoal. Be prepared to treat for shock. Late complications occur after a 2 to 5–day asymptomatic period and are caused by toxic injury resulting in liver, kidney, adrenal, and central nervous system damage.

Even with intensive care, the ingestion of one well-chewed seed can be fatal. Conversely, people who have eaten several unchewed seeds have experienced no illness.

# CANDLENUT
## *(Kukui) (Aleurites moluccana)*

Ancient Polynesian settlers introduced the candlenut tree, or *kukui*, to Hawai'i. Because people have spread these trees throughout the tropics for so long, it is difficult to tell where they originated. Today, *kukui* trees are conspicuous and common in Hawai'i's valley floors, where they flourish.

Even from a distance, *kukui* trees are easy to distinguish in a

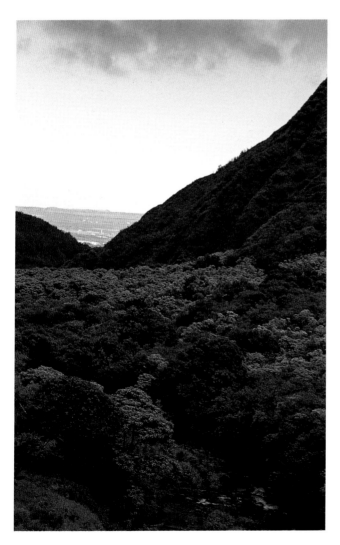

The candlenut tree is commonly called the *kukui* tree in Hawai'i. Pale hairs on the leaves give them a light green color, making the trees stand out in a forest. The *kukui* is Hawai'i's state tree. Contact with its sap can cause a rash. *(Craig Thomas)*

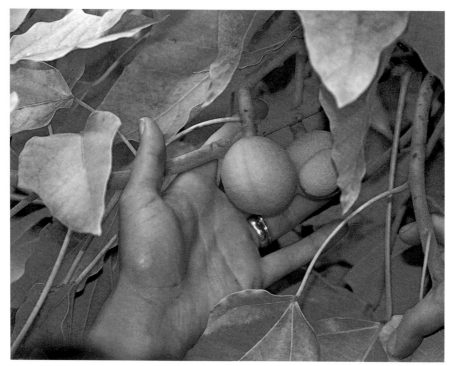

Eating raw *kukui* nuts causes vomiting and diarrhea. Once cooked, the nuts are safe to eat. Ancient Hawaiians used cooked *kukui* nuts as a relish. *(Susan Scott)*

forest. Downy, white hairs on *kukui* leaves give them a light green cast, and the pale green stands out from the darker trees around them. The scientific name for candlenut trees, *Aleurites,* derives from the pale appearance: the Greek word meaning floury.

Candlenut trees grow to about 60 feet tall. Small, white flowers produce the nuts for which the tree was named. The nuts are 50 percent oil. When eaten raw, they are poisonous.

# Toxin

The toxins in *kukui* are the irritants saponin and phorbol. These chemicals are found in all parts of the tree, but the raw seeds are usually the culprit in poisonings. Candlenut toxins are irritating to the skin, stomach, and intestines but are not medically dangerous except to small children or people with previous, serious illness.

Skin contact with the watery sap can cause a rash.

Cooking alters the toxins and makes the nuts safe to eat in small amounts.

## Traditional and Modern Uses

Ancient Hawaiians used nearly every part of the *kukui* tree. They extracted medicines from the flower, nuts, and bark for applying to cuts, boils, and fractures. Hawaiians rubbed candlenut oil on pregnant women's bellies to prevent stretch marks on the skin. They ate the nuts or oil raw for a laxative. Some Hawaiians and other Polynesians sometimes gargle with an infusion of *kukui* bark to treat thrush, mouth sores, and sore throats. Using any part of *kukui* as a remedy is scientifically unproven and may be harmful.

For light, ancient Hawaiians burned *kukui* nuts skewered on bamboo sticks (hence, the name candlenut). They also burned *kukui* oil for light. The bark and nuts were used to

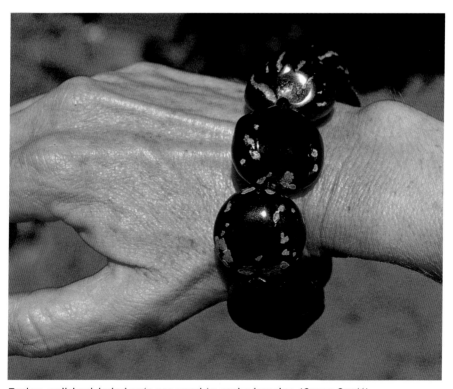

Today, polished *kukui* nuts are used to make jewelry. (*Susan Scott*)

make a black dye. *Kukui* wood was favored for making fish floats and canoe parts. When cooked, the nuts were eaten as a relish.

Today, people use *kukui* nuts for bracelets and *lei*. *Kukui* is the Hawai'i state tree.

## Incidence

Candlenuts are a moderate cause of illness or skin rash in Hawai'i. In 1997, the Hawaii Poison Center received calls from eight people reporting exposure to candlenuts; in 1998, thirteen people called. These numbers likely represent only a fraction of all *kukui* exposures experienced by Hawai'i residents and visitors.

## Signs and Symptoms

Contact with the watery sap of *kukui* trees can cause a red, itching skin rash.

People usually feel uncomfortable, warm, and nauseated shortly after eating raw *kukui* seeds. Vomiting, severe abdominal cramping, and diarrhea follows for about a day. Four seeds are enough to cause diarrhea.

 ## First Aid

For skin irritations, wash the area thoroughly with soap and water. For itching, try 1 percent hydrocortisone cream 4 times a day, and 1 or 2 25-milligram diphenhydramine (Benadryl) tablets every 6 hours. Diphenhydramine may cause drowsiness: Do not drive, swim, or surf after taking this medication. Give children diphenhydramine syrup, following the dosage directions on the package.

For diarrhea, drink water and wait. Diarrhea from *kukui* nuts usually disappears in a day or so on its own.

A physician should see children who have eaten raw *kukui* nuts. Adults with a persistent rash or persistent vomiting and/or diarrhea after eating these nuts should also consult a physician.

For facial swelling, any difficulty breathing, or collapse, call 911. Take the nuts to the emergency room for identification.

## Advanced Medical Treatment

No specific antidote or clinically useful diagnostic test exists for candlenut rash or poisoning. Most cases are self-limiting.

For ingestions, direct treatment at controlling emesis and diarrhea; replace fluids and electrolytes as needed.

# CASSAVA
## (Manihot esculenta)

Cassava, a bushy shrub native to Brazil, grows 3 to 9 feet tall. Other common names for cassava are tapioca and manioc.

Today, people throughout the subtropics and tropics, including Hawai'i, grow cassava in gardens for its edible roots.

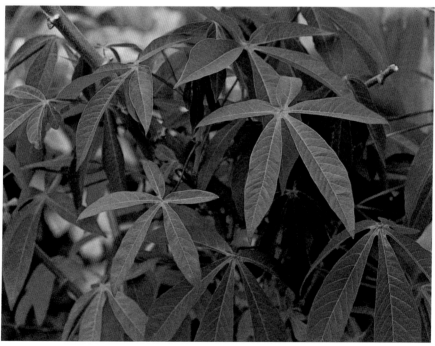

Some people grow cassava plants for their beauty rather than for food. The leaves are larger than a human hand and have red stems. Cassava leaves may be poisonous if eaten raw. *(Susan Scott)*

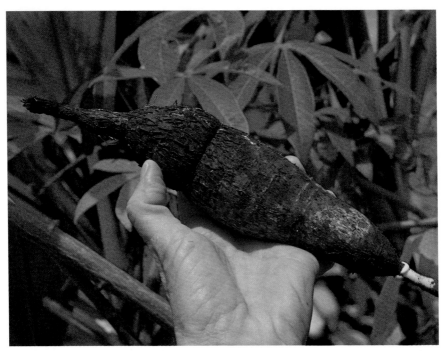

Cassava is usually cultivated for its root (pictured). The roots are edible only after thorough boiling. If eaten uncooked, cassava can cause cyanide poisoning. *(Susan Scott)*

Some varieties of cassava are harmless but others carry a deadly poison. Thorough cooking makes this poison harmless.

Some people grow cassava in gardens simply because the plants are beautiful. The leaves of this plant are 4 to 8 inches across.

## Toxin

Though the leaves of cassava may be poisonous, the highest concentration of poison is in its roots. Cassava toxins are the cyanogenic glycosides linamarin and lotaustralin. If eaten raw or undercooked, cyanogenic glycosides undergo a chemical change (hydrolysis) in the digestive tract that liberates potentially lethal hydrocyanic acid. This chemical process takes place slowly in an acid environment, as in the stomach, but takes place rapidly in an alkaline environment, as in the small intestine.

Cyanide is extremely toxic to humans because it renders the body's cells incapable of using oxygen.

## Traditional and Modern Uses

Cassava has been a food staple for centuries. Thoroughly boiled cassava roots, which resemble sweet potatoes, are eaten like potatoes (the water discarded).

Some people use the roots to make tapioca. To prepare tapioca, the cook crushes cassava root, adds water, mixes thoroughly, and allows the starch from the root to settle. The cook then removes any remaining root and boils the starch. Soon, the mixture forms the tiny, familiar balls known as tapioca.

## Incidence

Most people who grow cassava know of its poisonous potential when eaten raw or undercooked. Accidents are therefore rare. In 1997 and 1998, the Hawaii Poison Center received no calls from people about cassava poisoning.

## Signs and Symptoms

Because a chemical reaction must take place in the digestive tract before cyanide is released, the onset of symptoms may begin several hours after eating. Once the cyanide is formed, the victim at first feels dizzy and tired. Then, victims may have stomach pain, vomiting, weakness, and/or excessive sweating. Mucus membranes, nail beds, and skin may be bluish, but this sign is not always present in cyanide poisoning.

In severe poisonings, victims may have rapid, then slowed breathing, seizures, muscle weakness, loss of bladder control, and coma.

 ## First Aid

Because raw cassava can produce cyanide, regard eating any of it uncooked, or possibly undercooked, as a medical emergency. Go straight to the nearest emergency room. If symptoms have already begun, or if the victim has any difficulty breathing, call 911. Take roots and leaves of the plant to the emergency room for identification.

## Advanced Medical Treatment

If the patient is symptomatic, give charcoal. Victims require cardiac monitoring and 100 percent oxygen therapy.

For patients with significant symptoms, such as loss of consciousness, unstable vital signs, seizures, or acidosis, use the cyanide antidote kit.

Obtain baseline arterial blood gases, electrolytes, lactate, and cyanide levels. Do not delay therapy for results of cyanide testing. Monitor methemoglobin levels in patients receiving treatment from the kit. Dialysis after the kit treatment may improve acidosis and remove thiocyanate from the blood.

Chronic poisoning occurs in people eating cyanogenic diets and causes neuropathy with color blindness, deafness, spastic paraparesis, and ataxia. The seeds and pits of apples, apricots, cherries, peaches, plums, as well as lima beans and sorghum, contain cyanogenic glycosides. The crushed seeds of some of these are sold as "health foods," vitamin supplements, or cancer remedies.

# CASTOR BEAN
## (Ricinus communis)

The castor bean plant is native from east and northeast Africa to the Middle East but now grows throughout the world. This sprawling bush, from 3 to 30 feet tall, has been in Hawai'i at least since 1819 and has become a common weed in dry, disturbed areas, such as roadsides.

Castor bean plants have distinctive leaves, 4 to 30 inches wide with five to eleven points. The round fruit is covered with soft bristles; inside are three mottled brown, tick-shaped seeds called beans. People know these beans mainly for their oil. About 50 percent of the seed is castor oil.

Though sources vary, it is wise to regard all parts of this plant as poisonous. The coat of the castor bean is, without question, extremely poisonous. Powder from the beans can cause asthma and/or skin rashes.

Hawaiians have five interchangeable names for these plants: *pāʻaila, kolī, kaʻapehā, kamākou,* and *lāʻau ʻaila.*

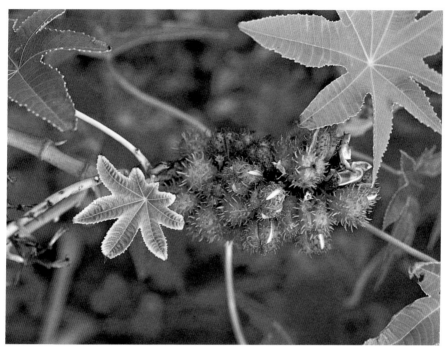

Castor bean plants are common roadside weeds in Hawai'i. The beans, inside these prickly hulls, contain an oil once commonly used as a powerful laxative. The seed coats on the beans contain ricin, one of the most toxic compounds known. Ricin is so toxic, one chewed seed can kill a child. *(Susan Scott)*

# Toxin

Castor bean plants, particularly the seed coats, contain a potentially lethal toxin known as ricin, a toxalbumin. Ricin is one of the most toxic compounds known.

Toxalbumins cause severe bleeding lesions in the mouth, esophagus, stomach, and intestines. The lesions are similar to alkaline burns, though the onset of toxalbumin lesions is delayed several hours after ingestion. Once absorbed into the bloodstream, toxalbumins interfere with cell function and cause cell damage, leading to serious liver, kidney, adrenal, and nerve damage.

Toxalbumins are so toxic that a single chewed bean can kill a child; eight to ten chewed beans can be lethal to an adult.

Because the seed coats on castor beans are hard, a person can survive unharmed if they swallow intact beans whole. Thus, the degree of poisoning a person experiences depends on how thoroughly the victim chewed the beans. People also can be poisoned if the toxin is absorbed through a cut or open sore. Even a needle prick while stringing beans in *lei* can cause serious poisoning.

Though not closely related scientifically to castor beans, black-eyed Susan seeds and species of *Jatropha* also carry toxalbumins.

The substance leftover in the seeds after oil has been expressed from castor beans is used to make a powdered fertilizer. It contains a protein allergen that in some people causes a rash, or when inhaled, causes asthmalike reactions.

## Traditional and Modern Uses

Egyptians four thousand years ago were expressing castor bean oil from the seeds of *Ricinus communis*. In Africa, people feed their silkworms castor bean leaves. Some Hawaiians rub castor bean leaves on the face to relieve fever.

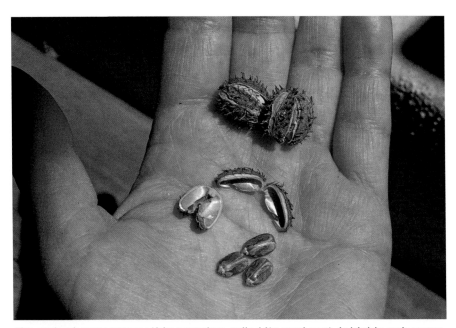

The castor bean's papery thin covering, called its seed coat, is highly poisonous. In this picture, the seed coats, still on the seeds, are brown with silvery marks (bottom). Above the seeds (center) are the hulls, also known as the plant's fruit. Intact fruits are pictured at top. *(Susan Scott)*

Using the castor bean plant as a remedy is scientifically unproven and may be harmful or even cause death.

Castor beans are the source of castor oil, the once common laxative. They are also used today in the manufacture of soap, margarine, lubricants, paints, inks, plastics, and linoleum.

In Ecuador, people string the seeds on sticks and light them like candles. In Hawai'i, castor beans are sometimes strung into *lei*. Ricin, the toxin in castor beans, has been used as a chemical warfare agent and is also a commercial mole (the animal) killer. Researchers have found promise in ricin as an anticancer drug.

A powder known as pomace remaining in the castor bean after the oil has been removed is used as fertilizer.

## Incidence

Though castor bean plants are plentiful in Hawai'i, exposures are uncommon, perhaps because most people are aware of the plant's extreme toxicity. In 1997, the Hawaii Poison Center received only one call from a person exposed to castor beans; no calls were recorded for 1998.

People in Hawai'i were not always aware of the dangers of this plant. Two soldiers died at Schofield Barracks in 1920 from eating castor beans as a laxative. Before 1944, a Hawai'i visitor nearly died from biting into a castor bean.

In 1978, a Bulgarian political exile in London died after an assassin stabbed him in the leg with a small, spherical capsule attached to the tip of an umbrella. The coroner said ricin was responsible for the death.

Children have died after eating two or three seeds; adults have died from as few as four. Six seeds have killed a horse.

People have become poisoned by pricking a finger while stringing castor beans in jewelry.

## Signs and Symptoms

Wheezing and difficulty breathing can develop in people exposed to the powdered fertilizer made from castor beans, or the burlap bags it comes in. Handling castor beans, or this fertilizer, can cause an allergic skin rash.

Pricking a finger while stringing castor beans can cause

immediate, painful swelling, a cold sweat, and throat and nasal congestion.

In the eyes, juice from these beans can cause redness, tearing and swelling, and loss of eye tissue, depending on the concentration.

After swallowing broken or chewed castor beans, people do not usually develop symptoms immediately; it may take anywhere from 2 hours to 3 days. Then, the victim has a burning sensation in the mouth and throat, followed by nausea, vomiting, and diarrhea, often with bleeding. In severe cases, open sores form in the mouth, esophagus, and throughout the stomach and intestines. These symptoms look like chemical burns. Blood in the urine is common.

Dehydration follows. Death occurs as a result of fluid loss.

## First Aid

For asthmalike symptoms or if a skin rash develops after handling castor bean products, consult a doctor. It may be simply an allergy, but because of the toxicity of castor beans, exposures warrant medical attention. Cases of poisoning by inhalation of ricin have been reported.

Getting castor bean toxin under the skin by a needle prick, in the eyes, or in the body by swallowing is always a medical emergency. Call 911. Take the beans, and the rest of the plant if available, to the emergency room for identification.

## Advanced Medical Treatment

No specific antidote or clinically useful diagnostic test exists for toxalbumin poisoning. Make the diagnosis by physical exam and history.

Either eaten or absorbed through a cut, this toxin is life threatening because of potential shock from fluid and electrolyte loss. Decontaminate exposed skin and eyes. Examine eyes with a slit lamp and perform funduscopic exam to check for both pupillary dilation and constriction. Retinal hemorrhage and optic neuritis have been reported.

Gastrointestinal injury is similar to caustic alkaline burns, though the onset is delayed 2 to 3 hours after ingestion.

Keep asymptomatic patients suspected of swallowing one or

more seeds under observation for at least 8 hours. Instruct care-givers to call 911 immediately if symptoms begin later at home.

For ingestions, give charcoal. Be prepared to treat for shock. Late complications occur after a 2 to 5–day asymptomatic period and are caused by toxic injury to the liver, kidneys, adrenal glands, and central nervous system.

Even with intensive care, the ingestion of one well-chewed seed can be fatal. Conversely, people who have eaten several unchewed seeds have experienced no illness.

Use standard treatment for asthmalike symptoms and allergic skin rash. These symptoms are from protein allergies, not the toxalbumin ricin.

# CERBERA
## (Cerbera manghas)

*Cerbera manghas* is a tree native to Australia, Southeast Asia, and some islands of Polynesia (but not Hawai'i). People in Hawai'i occasionally grow these trees for their abundant white, sweet-smelling flowers, similar to plumeria flowers but smaller. The fruits, 2 to 4 inches long, resemble mangoes but are extremely bitter. Branches of this tree contain a milky sap.

## Toxin

Cerbera trees contain the cardiac glycoside cerberin. Cardiac glycosides block normal electrical impulses throughout the body, including the heart, by interfering with the exchange of sodium and potassium in and out of nerve and muscle cells.

People experience a wide range of responses after eating plants containing cardiac glycosides. Some barely become sick; others have died. Regard all parts of this plant, whether green, dry, or burning, as extremely toxic. Never use a cerbera stick to roast marshmallows or hot dogs and do not cook food over a cerbera-wood fire.

Sap from this tree can irritate eyes and skin. Inhaling plant

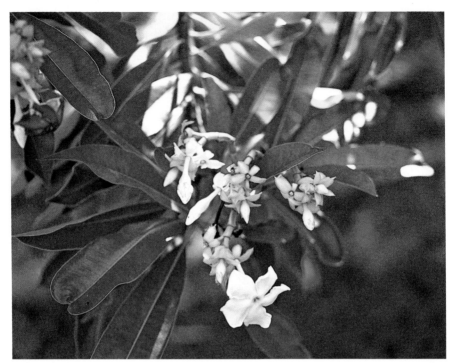

Cerbera flowers have a shape similar to plumeria flowers, only smaller. These cerbera flowers are about 2 inches across. All parts of cerbera trees contain a powerful heart toxin and are extremely poisonous. *(Susan Scott)*

dust while raking cerbera leaves may irritate the nose and throat. Inhaling smoke from burning cerbera trees may cause poisoning.

## Traditional and Modern Uses

Fishermen in the Philippines use the seeds of cerbera trees to stun fish. People there also use oil from the seeds as a medicine applied to the skin. They sometimes eat the bark, leaves, and milky sap to induce vomiting and as a laxative. Home remedies using cerbera are scientifically unproven, dangerous, and may cause death.

A close relative of *Cerbera manghas* is *C. tanghin*. This tree, rare in Hawaiʻi, is much more poisonous than *C. manghas*. People from East Africa and Madagascar once used the sap as an arrow poison and the seeds in ordeal trials. If the accused survived the ordeal of eating some of the poisonous seeds, they were judged innocent of the offense in question; if they died, they were presumed to have been guilty.

## Incidence

Cerbera trees are rare in Hawai'i gardens and do not grow wild in the Islands. In 1997 and 1998, the Hawaii Poison Center received no calls from people with cerbera exposure. Because its attractive fruit contains a potentially lethal toxin, however, the cerbera tree warrants attention. Poisonings may occur from people mistaking the fruits for mangoes.

## Signs and Symptoms

Inhaling cerbera leaf dust can cause sneezing or coughing. Skin contact with cerbera leaves can cause a red, itching rash. Sap in the eyes can cause tearing and redness.

Swallowing any part of a cerbera tree, particularly the fruit, can cause nausea, vomiting, abdominal pain, and cramping.

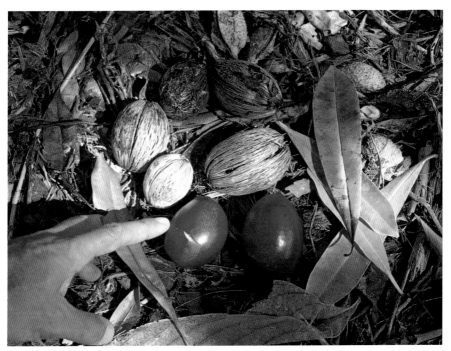

The ripe fruits of cerbera trees look like mangoes but taste extremely bitter. This is fortunate because eating the fruits can kill a person. *(Susan Scott)*

This discomfort can last for several hours before generalized heart symptoms begin, including slow or irregular heartbeat, dizziness, headache, and confusion. Victims may feel drowsy or giddy.

## First Aid

Thoroughly wash skin exposed to sap of this tree with soap and water. Rinse exposed eyes for at least 15 minutes with tap water. For persistent itching, blurred vision, or violent coughing after raking leaves, consult a doctor.

Regard as a medical emergency the swallowing of any part of this tree, the inhaling of smoke from it, or the eating of food cooked on its branches. Call 911. Take fruit, flowers, and a branch from the tree to the emergency room for identification.

## Advanced Medical Treatment

The effects of the cardiac glycocide cerberin are similar to digoxin and digitoxin. Therefore, laboratory tests for these drugs may be positive for some (but not all) cerbera poisonings. Because these tests rely on cross-reactivity between the plant's cardiac glycoside and digoxin or digitoxin, serum levels do not necessarily correlate with biological activity. A low digoxin or digitoxin level may indicate a potentially fatal level of cerbera cardiac glycoside.

An elevated potassium level in the presence of a plant ingestion suggests cardiac glycoside exposure.

If the patient has swallowed cerbera an hour or less before going to the ER, empty the stomach. For all patients suspected of eating cerbera, regardless of time elapsed, give charcoal.

Victims suspected of eating plants containing cardiac glycosides require cardiac monitoring. The effect of cardiac glycosides on the heart, however, may be delayed; monitor asymptomatic patients for at least 12 hours before discharge.

For life-threatening arrythmias, hyperkalemia, prolonged PR intervals, widened QRS segments, or altered mental status, administer 10 vials of digoxin immune FAB intravenously. In one case of cardiac glycoside poisoning from oleander, the patient woke up 4 minutes after FAB treatment was started, and his potassium level normalized in an hour. If improvement is minimal, give another 10 vials. The cross-reactivity for binding may require a high concentration of digoxin immune FAB.

The risks of digoxin immune FAB include fever, apnea, hypokalemia, and hypoglycemia. Rebound toxicity occurs in 3 to 11 days in a small fraction of patients treated with digoxin immune FAB. Some researchers suggest a continuous FAB infusion after an initial bolus. Hemoperfusion and forced diuresis are of no benefit.

If FAB is not available, use IV atropine to treat bradycardia, and use lidocaine, amiodarone, or phenytoin for ventricular arrythmias. Consider phenytoin or a pacemaker in victims with second- or third-degree heart block.

# CESTRUM
## (*Cestrum* species)

Cestrums are small shrubs and trees native to Central and South America. People grow night-blooming cestrum (*Cestrum nocturnum*) for its fragrant scent, which is more powerful at night than by day. The Hawaiian name for the plant, *'alaaumoe*, means fragrance late at night. This cestrum bears greenish white flowers and white berries.

The closely related day cestrum (*Cestrum diurnum*) is fragrant during the day. It has white flowers and black berries. Another relative, the orange cestrum (*C. aurantiacum*), produces orange flowers that smell strongest in the daytime.

These three cestrum plants were introduced to Hawai'i before 1871. Today, they grow in gardens, yards, and in the wild.

Cestrum berries are poisonous to eat.

## Toxin

When unripe, cestrum berries produce solanine, a glycoalkaloid toxin. Solanine damages the lining of the digestive tract and can also depress the central nervous system, thus slowing the heart rate and lowering blood pressure.

When ripe, cestrum berries produce an anticholinergic toxin

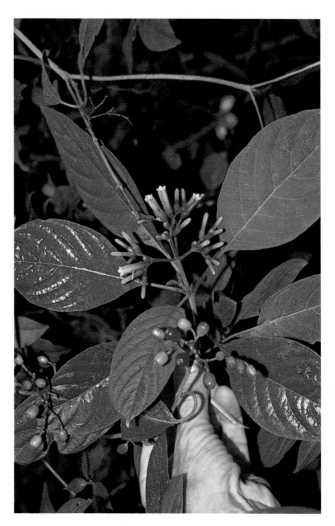

This cestrum (*Cestrum aurantiacum*) produces orange flowers, which smell strongest during the day. Other cestrums in Hawai'i have white flowers, with scents strongest either during the day or at night, depending on the species. Some people feel ill after smelling cestrums. *(Susan Scott)*

that resembles atropine. Like atropine, this toxin also affects the central nervous system.

Rarely, both toxins are present, which can lead to confusing and contradictory symptoms, appearing one after another. For example, solanine can cause people to salivate excessively, but the atropine-like toxin causes dry mouth.

## Traditional and Modern Uses

In tropical America, healers use the fruit and sap of night cestrum to treat epilepsy. This treatment is scientifically unproven and may be harmful.

In Hawaiʻi, *lei* makers sometimes use these sweet-smelling flowers in *lei*.

## Incidence

Cestrums do not bear abundant fruits, and poisonings from them are rare. In 1997 and 1998, the Hawaii Poison Center received no calls from people with cestrum exposure.

The strong odor of night cestrum has made some people ill.

## Signs and Symptoms

Most people enjoy the scent of night cestrum, but some people suffer headache, nausea, dizziness, and weakness after smelling the flowers in full bloom.

Rubbing one or both eyes after handling this plant may cause the pupil(s) to dilate. This causes sensitivity to bright light and blurred vision, which can last for about a week.

Symptoms of solanine poisoning from eating unripe berries are mainly nausea, vomiting, headache, and diarrhea. Sometimes, the victim has excessive salivation. Most of these symptoms begin within 2 to 24 hours and last 3 to 6 days.

Symptoms of atropine-like poisoning from eating ripe cestrum berries include warm skin, dilated pupils (with blurred vision, and sensitivity to bright light), dry mouth (causing difficulty swallowing and speaking), reddening of the face, restlessness, irritability, disorientation, hallucinations, and/or delirium.

Blurred vision and dilated pupils from eating cestrum berries may last 7 to 12 days.

In severe poisonings, victims may feel cold, may be agitated and combative, may be unable to urinate, may have seizures, paralysis, coma, respiratory failure, circulation collapse, and may die.

To remember the varied signs and symptoms of atropine intoxication, medical doctors traditionally memorize the following phrase: "Hot as a hare, blind as a bat, dry as a bone, red as a beet, and mad as a hatter."

 ## First Aid

Wash hands thoroughly after handling cestrum flowers or leaves. Rinse exposed eyes with copious amounts of tap water. For persistent blurred vision, consult a doctor.

Mild to moderate cases of cestrum poisoning disappear overnight without treatment.

For persistent vomiting and diarrhea, or combative behavior, go to an emergency room. For facial swelling, any difficulty breathing, or collapse, call 911. Take flowers, branches, leaves, and berries to the emergency room for identification.

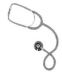

## Advanced Medical Treatment

No specific antidote or clinically useful diagnostic test exists for cestrum poisoning, which is easily mistaken for bacterial gastroenteritis. Make the diagnosis by physical exam and history. Use antiemetics as needed. Replace fluids and electrolytes. Atropine may be needed for symptomatic bradycardia.

Cestrum poisoning may also present as atropine poisoning. Atropine impairs peristalsis. Therefore, in severe poisonings, consider emptying the stomach even if more than an hour has elapsed since ingestion. For all ingestions, give charcoal. Catheterize for urinary retention. Use diazepam as necessary for sedation.

Consider physostigmine only for uncontrollable hyperthermia, supraventricular tachycardia with hemodynamic instability, therapy-resistant seizures, and extreme delirium. The recommended dose of physostigmine in adults is 1 to 2 milligrams intravenously over 5 minutes. Repeat every 15 minutes as needed. Never exceed 4 mg in 30 minutes.[1]

For children, start with 0.02 milligrams per kilogram, increasing dose as necessary to 0.5 mg. Repeat as needed to control symptoms. Maximum dose is 2 mg.[2]

Physostigmine dramatically reverses coma and other anticholinergic symptoms but may mask solanine symptoms in mixed poisonings. Physostigmine may also cause seizures. Never use physostigmine just to keep a patient awake.

# CHINABERRY
## (Melia azedarach)

The chinaberry tree, native to tropical Asia, was introduced to Hawai'i probably as early as 1839. Today, besides growing in

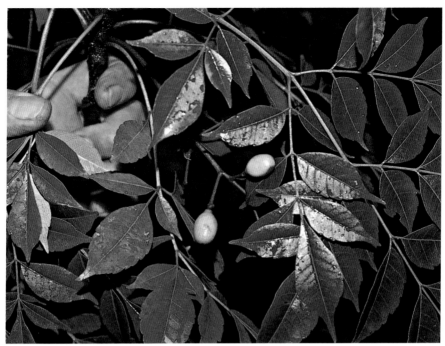

The small, golden fruits of the chinaberry tree taste terrible, a good feature because eating them can cause death. *(Susan Scott)*

gardens and parks, these trees grow wild in gulches and pastures. Chinaberry trees grow to 60 feet tall, with wide-spreading branches. Their Hawaiian name is ʻinia.

People plant chinaberry trees for shade and for their sweet-smelling lavender flowers, blooming from March to June. The fruits are golden half-inch balls, which hang from the tree throughout the fall and winter, even after the leaves have fallen. These fruits are bitter-tasting and nauseating, a fortunate feature because they can be highly poisonous if eaten.

## Toxin

All parts of the chinaberry tree contain several alkaloids called tetranortriterpene neurotoxins. These toxins inhibit an insect hormone that allows insects to molt. Thus, insect larvae cannot mature on this tree. In humans, the toxins attack the central nervous system.

Chinaberry trees also contain an unknown toxin that damages the human digestive system when any part of the tree is swallowed.

The fruit is particularly toxic, but the leaves, bark, flowers, and roots of this plant may also be toxic. Yellow, ripe fruits are more toxic than green, unripe ones.

The toxicity of chinaberry trees varies greatly with region and growing conditions. To be safe, regard all parts of this tree as potentially lethal.

## Traditional and Modern Uses

On Maui, people once used chinaberry tea to bathe wounds on victims of Hansen's disease (leprosy). Chinaberry has been used as folk medicine in southwest Asia to treat worms, constipation, and menstrual cramps, sometimes with lethal results. Use of any part of the chinaberry tree as a remedy is scientifically unproven and extremely dangerous, possibly resulting in death.

A chemical in chinaberry fruit and leaves repels some insects and prevents others from molting. Because of this, some people

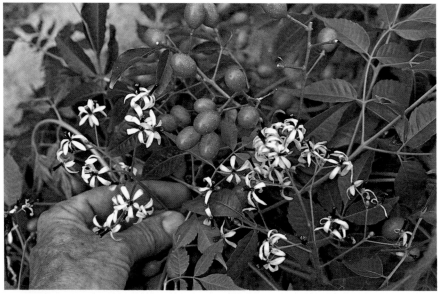

Chinaberry trees bloom in the spring, bearing small lavender flowers with a pleasant scent. Green chinaberry fruits (pictured) usually are less toxic than the ripe yellow fruits, but it is wise to regard all parts of this tree as highly poisonous during all stages of their growth. *(Susan Scott)*

use chinaberry leaves and fruit to ward off insects while drying or storing edible fruits. Ground chinaberry fruits are used as insecticides and flea powder.

Fishermen sometimes use the bark of this tree to stun fish.

## Incidence

In 1997 and 1998, the Hawaii Poison Center received no calls from people with chinaberry exposure.

Poisoning from chinaberry fruit in humans is rare because of the fruit's bitter, nauseating taste. Early in this century, however, a three-year-old girl in Argentina died after eating an unknown number of fruits. An East Indian girl died after eating six to eight fruits.

Poisonings occur most often through folk remedies, when people drink tea made from chinaberry leaves or bark. In Singapore, an eighteen-year-old woman died three days after drinking chinaberry tea for menstrual cramps.

Pigs are particularly susceptible to chinaberry poisoning, and other types of livestock also have been killed from eating parts of this tree.

## Signs and Symptoms

Intense vomiting, abdominal pain, and diarrhea usually occur a few hours after eating chinaberry. Victims become intensely thirsty and may be cold, pale, and sweaty.

As the toxin progresses, victims may have dilated pupils, grind their teeth, and be unable to talk. Parts of the body may become paralyzed, sometimes causing difficulty breathing. Lips and nail beds may turn blue. Seizures and coma follow. Death from respiratory failure can occur 12 to 24 hours after symptoms begin.

 ## First Aid

Regard as a medical emergency the eating of any part of a chinaberry tree. Even if the victim shows no symptoms, drive him or her immediately to the nearest emergency room. If symptoms have begun, or if the victim has any difficulty breathing, call 911. Take fruit and a branch of the tree (with leaves) to the emergency room for identification.

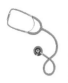

## Advanced Medical Treatment

No antidote or diagnostic test exists for chinaberry ingestion. Symptoms vary widely from case to case, depending on what part of the plant was eaten and where it was growing.

Direct treatment at controlling emesis. Give charcoal; replace fluids and electrolytes as needed.

Rarely, patients have altered levels of consciousness; be prepared to treat seizures and to protect the airway.

Because autopsy of poisoned animals shows fatty degeneration of the liver, get baseline liver function tests.

# CROWN FLOWER
## (Calotropis gigantea)

Crown flowers are native throughout tropical and subtropical regions of Africa, Asia, and the Caribbean Islands but are now pantropical. These large shrubs, members of the milkweed family, grow about 15 feet tall and bear lavender or white flowers.

In Hawai'i, people cultivate these bushes for the flowers. The bushes are now common throughout the Islands.

Crown flowers were a favorite of Hawaiian Queen Lili'uokalani. Their Hawaiian name is *pua kalaunu.*

## Toxin

The white, milky sap from this plant contains calcium oxalate and an enzyme that breaks down proteins. These substances cause irritation when squirted or rubbed into the eye but do not cause permanent vision damage.

Crown flower sap also contains a substance that causes a local allergic reaction in some people. Most people who get the sap on their skin, though, have no reaction to it. Those who do are allergic to this particular substance.

Inhaling plant dust while raking crown flower leaves may irritate the nose and throat.

All parts of the crown flower plant contain calotropin, a cardiac glycoside. Cardiac glycosides block normal electrical

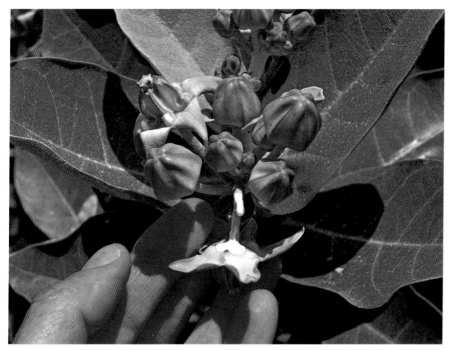

Crown flowers are either white or lavender. Some (but not all) people are allergic to the sap of these plants. Swallowing any part of this plant is extremely dangerous because the entire plant contains a powerful heart toxin. *(Susan Scott)*

impulses throughout the body, including the heart, by interfering with the exchange of sodium and potassium in and out of nerve and muscle cells.

People experience a wide range of responses after eating plants containing cardiac glycosides. Some barely become sick; others have died. Regard all parts of this plant, either green or dried, as extremely toxic if eaten. Inhaling smoke from burning crown flower bushes may cause poisoning.

## Traditional and Modern Uses

People in India use crown flower leaves as poultices. For fevers, they swallow small amounts of the bark, leaves, and roots. These traditional uses are scientifically unproven, extremely dangerous, and can even cause death.

Crown flower fruits, which do not usually develop in Hawai'i, are full of fluff used in India as pillow stuffing. Indians also use crown flowers as an ingredient in gunpowder and the bark fibers for fishlines.

## Incidence

In 1997, the Hawaii Poison Center received calls from eleven people with crown flower exposures; in 1998, nine people called. These numbers likely represent only a fraction of the number of crown flower exposures experienced by Hawai'i residents and visitors.

*Lei* makers sometimes get the sap of these flowers squirted into their eyes when stringing or picking the flowers. People who are allergic to the sap can develop a rash from wearing a crown flower *lei*. An allergic person may develop a rash from the second, or any subsequent, contact with crown flowers. The first exposure causes sensitivity, and subsequent exposures cause a rash.

Rarely do people or animals eat the sap or flowers from this plant, because of the bitter taste.

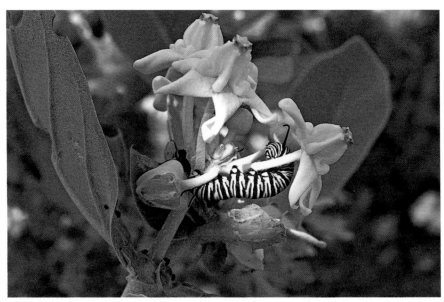

Crown flower bushes are a favorite food of the caterpillar of the monarch butterfly. The caterpillars apparently are not harmed by the plant's cardiac toxin, potentially lethal to humans. *(Susan Scott)*

# Signs and Symptoms

People who are allergic to crown flower sap may have red, itchy bumps around the neck or on the hands after wearing a crown flower *lei*.

In the eye, crown flower sap immediately causes a burning sensation plus redness, intense tearing, and swelling of the eyelid. Sometimes these symptoms disappear within an hour, but the sensation of something-in-the-eye and blurry vision remains. This blurring can persist for 5 to 7 days.

People who eat any part of the crown flower plant may have immediate burning, redness, and swelling of the lips and mouth.

Swallowing this plant can cause the victim to have nausea, vomiting, abdominal pain, and cramping. This can go on for several hours before the generalized heart symptoms begin. These are slow or irregular heartbeat, dizziness, headache, and confusion. Victims may feel drowsy or giddy.

## First Aid

Thoroughly wash skin exposed to crown flower sap with soap and water. For itching, try 1 percent hydrocortisone cream 4 times a day, and 1 or 2 25-milligram diphenhydramine (Benadryl) tablets every 6 hours. Diphenhydramine may cause drowsiness: Do not drive, swim, or surf after taking this medication. Give children diphenhydramine syrup, following the dosage directions on the package.

Rinse eyes exposed to crown flower sap for at least 15 minutes with tap water. For blurred vision, hives, or persistent skin redness go to an emergency room.

Regard as a medical emergency the swallowing of any part of this plant. Call 911. Take branches, leaves, and flowers of the plant to the emergency room for identification.

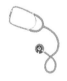

## Advanced Medical Treatment

The effects of the cardiac glycocides found in crown flower plants are similar to digoxin and digitoxin. Therefore, laboratory tests for these drugs may be positive for some (but not all) crown flower poisonings. Because these tests rely on cross-reactivity between the plant's cardiac glycosides and digoxin or digitoxin, serum levels do not necessarily correlate with biological activity. A low digoxin or digitoxin level may indicate a potentially fatal level of crown flower cardiac glycosides.

An elevated potassium level in the presence of a plant ingestion suggests cardiac glycoside exposure.

If the patient has swallowed crown flower an hour or less before going to the ER, empty the stomach. For all patients suspected of eating crown flower, regardless of time elapsed, give charcoal.

Victims suspected of eating plants containing cardiac glycosides require cardiac monitoring. However, the effect of cardiac glycosides on the heart may be delayed; monitor asymptomatic patients for at least 12 hours before discharge.

For life-threatening arrythmias, hyperkalemia, prolonged PR intervals, widened QRS segments, or altered mental status, administer 10 vials of digoxin immune FAB intravenously. In one case of cardiac glycoside poisoning from oleander, the patient woke up 4 minutes after FAB treatment was begun, and his potassium level normalized in an hour. If improvement is minimal, give another 10 vials. The cross-reactivity for binding may require a high concentration of digoxin immune FAB.

The risks of digoxin immune FAB include fever, apnea, hypokalemia, and hypoglycemia. Rebound toxicity occurs in 3 to 11 days in a small fraction of patients treated with digoxin immune FAB. Some researchers suggest a continuous FAB infusion after an initial bolus. Hemoperfusion and forced diuresis are of no benefit.

If FAB is not available, use IV atropine to treat bradycardia, and use lidocaine, amiodarone, or phenytoin for ventricular arrythmias. Consider phenytoin or a pacemaker in victims with second- or third-degree heart block.

No specific treatment exists for crown flower dermatitis.

In crown flower eye exposures, the cornea may be cloudy. Irrigate the eye thoroughly, examine with a slit lamp, then instill topical steroids.

# CUP OF GOLD AND SILVER CUP
## (*Solandra* species)

People grow the cup of gold plant *(Solandra maxima)* for its lovely large, yellow flowers, which measure 6 inches across. Inside the flowers, five distinctive purple lines radiate from the center. Cup of gold flowers, native to Mexico, Central America, and northern South America, are common throughout Hawai'i.

A close relative of cup of gold is silver cup *(Solandra grandiflora)*, native to Jamaica and Puerto Rico. These plants produce enormous flowers similar to cup of gold except they are white.

Both these flowers, which bloom in January, February, and March, have a strong, unusual smell. They also contain toxins.

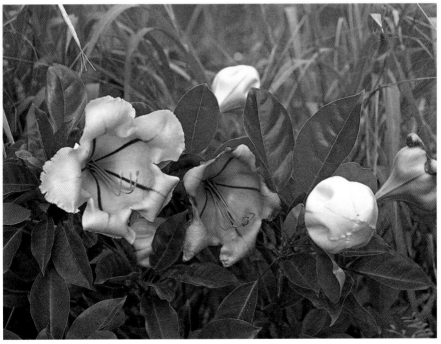

These cup of gold flowers are at various stages of growth. The older flowers are rust colored. At all stages, the flowers contain at least one, and sometimes two, toxins that effect the central nervous system. (*Susan Scott*)

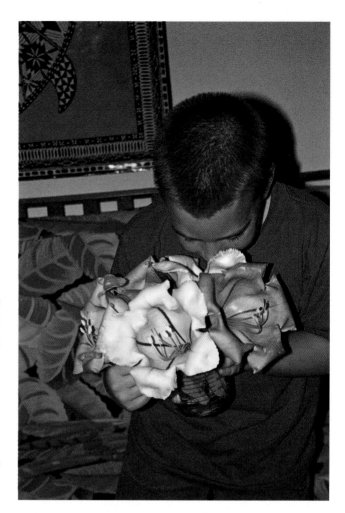

Cup of gold flowers have a strong scent pleasant to most people. Some people feel slightly ill after sniffing these flowers deeply. This boy had no symptoms after smelling the flowers repeatedly. *(Susan Scott)*

## Toxin

Both cup of gold and silver cup contain either the glyco-alkaloid toxin solanine, or atropine. Solanine damages the lining of the digestive tract and can also depress the central nervous system, thus slowing the heart rate and lowering blood pressure. Atropine also affects the central nervous system.

Rarely, both toxins are present, which can lead to confusing and contradictory symptoms, appearing one after another. For example, solanine can cause people to salivate excessively, but the atropine-like toxin causes dry mouth.

# Traditional and Modern Uses

In the past, the Aztec people of Mexico used these flowers to induce sacred hallucinations.

Some people today eat cup of gold or drink tea made from it to get high. This practice is extremely dangerous and could cause death.

# Incidence

Cup of gold and silver cup poisonings are rare in Hawai'i. In 1997 and 1998, the Hawaii Poison Center received no calls from people with exposure to these plants.

In Florida, several teen-agers became ill after eating cup of gold flowers or drinking tea made from the flowers. They recovered.

A mother accidentally poisoned her four-year-old asthmatic boy by giving him cup of gold tea. Someone had convinced her the tea would cure her son's asthma. The boy recovered.

A child suffered a headache and a temporarily dilated pupil after sniffing a cup of gold flower. Presumably, part of the flower touched his eye.

# Signs and Symptoms

Most people enjoy the smell of cup of gold and silver cup, but some people suffer headache, nausea, dizziness, and weakness after smelling them when the flowers are in full bloom.

Rubbing one or both eyes after handling this plant may cause the pupil(s) to dilate. This causes sensitivity to bright light and blurred vision, which can last for about a week.

Symptoms of solanine poisoning from eating or drinking tea from cup of gold or silver cup flowers are usually nausea, vomiting, headache, and diarrhea. Sometimes, the victim has excessive salivation. Most of these symptoms begin within 2 to 24 hours and last for 3 to 6 days.

Symptoms of atropine-like poisoning from eating these flowers, or drinking tea made from them, include warm skin, dilated pupils (causing blurred vision and sensitivity to bright light), dry mouth (causing difficulty swallowing and speaking), reddening of the face, restlessness, irritability, disorientation, hallucinations, and/or delirium.

Blurred vision and dilated pupils from eating these flowers can last for 7 to 12 days.

In severe poisonings, victims may feel cold, may be agitated and combative, may be unable to urinate, may have seizures, paralysis, coma, respiratory failure, circulation collapse, and may die.

To remember the varied signs and symptoms of this class of drug intoxication, medical doctors traditionally memorize the following phrase: "Hot as a hare, blind as a bat, dry as a bone, red as a beet, and mad as a hatter."

 ## First Aid

Wash hands thoroughly after handling cup of gold or silver cup flowers or leaves. Rinse exposed eyes with copious amounts of tap water. For persistent blurred vision, consult a doctor.

Mild to moderate cases of cup of gold or silver cup poisoning disappear overnight without treatment.

For hives or persistent vomiting and diarrhea, go to an emergency room. For facial swelling, any difficulty breathing, or collapse, call 911. Take flowers and leaves of the plant to the emergency room for identification.

 ## Advanced Medical Treatment

No specific antidote or clinically useful diagnostic test exists for cup of gold or silver cup poisoning, which appears either as gastroenteritis and/or atropine poisoning. Make the diagnosis by physical exam and history. Use antiemetics as needed. Replace fluids and electrolytes. Atropine may be needed for symptomatic bradycardia.

Poisoning from these plants may also present as atropine poisoning. Atropine impairs peristalsis. Therefore, in severe poisonings consider emptying the stomach even if more than one hour has elapsed since ingestion. For all ingestions, give charcoal. Catheterize for urinary retention. Use diazepam as necessary for sedation.

Consider physostigmine only for uncontrollable hyperthermia, supraventricular tachycardia with hemodynamic instability, therapy-resistant seizures, and extreme delirium. The recommended dose of physostigmine in adults is 1 to 2 milligrams intravenously over 5 minutes. Repeat every 15 minutes as needed. Never exceed 4 mg in 30 minutes.[1]

For children, start with 0.02 milligrams per kilogram, increasing dose as necessary to 0.5 mg. Repeat as needed to control symptoms. Maximum dose is 2 mg.[2]

Physostigmine dramatically reverses coma and other anti-cholinergic symptoms but may mask solanine symptoms in mixed poisonings. Physostigmine may also cause seizures. Never use physostigmine just to keep a patient awake.

# DUMB CANE
## (*Dieffenbachia* species)

Dumb canes are popular house and garden plants that are natives of tropical America. They grow well outdoors in shady spots and indoors as potted plants. They are easily prop-agated by stem cuttings, which root easily. Dumb cane plants are extremely common, growing in millions of American homes and offices. In Hawai'i, they are a common garden plant.

All dumb cane stems and leaves contain a juice highly irri-tating to the mouth, eyes, and sometimes to the skin.

## Toxin

All parts of all dieffenbachias contain calcium oxalate needles inside special cells of the plant. When broken, these cells shoot their needles for a distance of two or three cell lengths. This mechanical release causes traumatic injury to skin and mucus membranes. The resulting injury is far more severe than from other plants bearing calcium oxalate crystals. In fact, dieffenbachias have fewer calcium oxalate crystals than spinach, which is harmless when eaten raw. Researchers believe dieffenbachia needles also carry chemical toxins, probably protein-damaging enzymes, on their surfaces and in their grooves. Therefore, dieffenbachia needles act like tiny poison darts.

Feeding dieffenbachia juice to both male and female labora-tory rats makes them temporarily sterile.

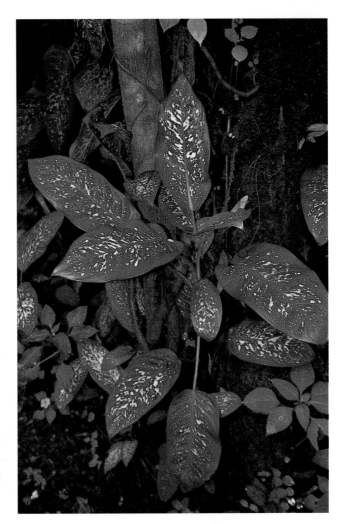

Dumb cane is named for its toxin. The plant touched to the mouth can cause such a severe reaction that a person becomes unintelligible or unable to speak. *(Susan Scott)*

## Traditional and Modern Uses

Native Amazonians combined dumb cane with curare to use in making poison arrows. In the Caribbean Islands, men once chewed dumb cane in the belief that it would make them sterile. People also have used dieffenbachia as medicine to treat gout, dropsy, sexual impotence, and sexual frigidity. These home remedies using this plant are scientifically unproven and may be extremely harmful.

The Nuremberg Trials after World War II revealed that

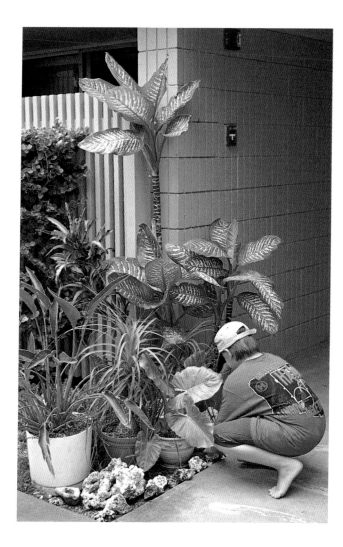

Because dumb cane grows well in low light, it is a common decorative plant in restaurants, offices, and shady gardens. When the plants are within easy reach, like these, they can be dangerous to young children. *(Susan Scott)*

Nazi doctors experimented with the sterilization effects of dieffenbachia on concentration camp prisoners. Equally abhorrent was the practice of rubbing dieffenbachia into the mouths of slaves as punishment in eighteenth-century Jamaica.

## Incidence

Because dumb cane is such a common house and garden plant, hundreds of children are poisoned by it each year in the United

States. Most are under the age of five and most recover. Three child deaths, though, have been reported in Brazil.

In 1997, the Hawaii Poison Center received calls from five people exposed to dieffenbachia; in 1998, seven people called. These numbers represent only a fraction of the number of dumb cane exposures experienced by Hawaiʻi residents and visitors.

# Signs and Symptoms

Some people develop burning, itching, and red bumps, sometimes with blisters, from handling dumb cane plants. The burning sensation may last up to 24 hours.

Dumb cane juice in the eye can cause immediate pain, sensitivity to light, swollen eyelids, spasms of the eyelids, and tearing. Vision may be blurred from swelling and inflammation of the surface of the eye. Eye symptoms are temporary but can last for three to four months.

Merely touching a piece of cut dumb cane to the mouth can cause tingling, pain, and an open sore. Blisters and peeling may form at the site of contact. Blisters usually last 5 to 10 days. Even such minor contact can render the victim unable to speak or make their speech unintelligible; hence, the common name dumb cane.

Biting and chewing a leaf or stem of dumb cane can cause mild to severe pain in the mouth immediately. This is sometimes followed by swelling of the tongue, lips, and mucus membranes inside the mouth. In severe cases, the tongue swells so much it protrudes from the mouth for up to three days. Because the vocal cords may become temporarily paralyzed, the victim may be unable to speak. Profuse salivation is common.

If swelling is severe in the mouth and throat, the victim may have difficulty breathing.

Vomiting and diarrhea is rare from this plant because the painful mouth symptoms begin before victims swallow much of the plant.

 First Aid

Rinse eyes exposed to dumb cane with tap water for 15 minutes. Wash exposed skin thoroughly with soap and water.

If pain, swelling, tearing, and blurring of vision continue after the rinse, or if the rash persists, consult a doctor.

Biting or chewing on a dieffenbachia leaf can result in only mild symptoms or can become a medical emergency. For a mild burning sensation without swelling, rinse the mouth with water or milk. For pain relief, try sucking on ice cubes or a Popsicle. Do not swallow the rinse solution, ice water, or melted Popsicle.

If there is any question about whether a child chewed on dieffenbachia, take the child to an emergency room. Children usually begin screaming and crying seconds after contact. If the tongue, lips, or mouth are swollen, call 911. Take leaves and stems of the plant to the emergency room for identification.

## Advanced Medical Treatment

No antidote or diagnostic test exists for dieffenbachia poisoning. The toxicity of these plants is extremely variable. The more the plant is chewed, the worse the symptoms.

Examine exposed eyes with a slit lamp for calcium oxalate crystals embedded in the cornea. Dexamethasone eye drops have been used to treat eye exposures, and the crystals gradually disappeared in two to three months. Whether the dexamethasone influenced the recovery is unknown.

Neither systemic steroids nor antihistamines have been shown to relieve the rash caused by this plant. Therefore, they are probably not useful topically for dieffenbachia skin rashes.

For ingestions, charcoal is not usually necessary, because victims swallow very little, if any, of this plant.

Death from eating this plant is rare but can occur from airway obstruction due to edema of the tongue, vocal cords, and esophagus. One patient required a tracheostomy for extreme tongue swelling. Be prepared to protect the airway.

Direct treatment at reducing pain and swelling. Viscous lidocaine may help relieve pain, but use it judiciously to avoid lidocaine toxicity. Narcotics may be necessary in severe cases.

# ELEPHANT EAR
## (*Alocasia* and *Xanthosoma* species)

Several species of plants common in Hawai'i are called elephant ears. They are named for their large, heart-shaped or spade-shaped leaves, which range from about 1 to 4 feet long. Elephant ears are close relatives of taro; their leaves have a family resemblance.

Some elephant ears growing in Hawai'i today come from tropical America and the Caribbean Islands. Others are from India, Sri Lanka, Southeast Asia, and Polynesia. One species (*Alocasia macrorrhizos*) was brought to Hawai'i by ancient Polynesian settlers as food to be eaten during times of famine. Named 'ape in Hawaiian, this species grows wild along streams or in other wet areas. Today, there are several other elephant ear species also named 'ape.

Elephant ears are common throughout Hawai'i and Florida, both indoors and out. In colder climates, the smaller ones are popular houseplants.

Like taro, some kinds of elephant ears have starchy roots, edible only after being cooked. People in some parts of Africa, Asia, the tropical Americas, and the Caribbean Islands regularly eat these roots; others reserve them for famine food.

## Toxin

All parts of the elephant ear plant contain bundles of needle-like calcium oxalate crystals. Some researchers believe that irritating proteins or a toxic alkaloid may also be present in these plants.

Calcium oxalate is a nonabsorbable salt of oxalic acid, a colorless, crystalline, potentially poisonous, organic acid found in many common food plants, such as spinach, rhubarb, tomatoes, grapes, and sweet potatoes. The human body produces its own oxalic acid. Some kidney stones contain calcium oxalate.

Whether eating calcium oxalate crystals is harmful depends on cooking methods and its concentration in a particular plant. Some plants bearing this substance require no cooking, others require considerable cooking, and some cannot be made edible by any amount of cooking.

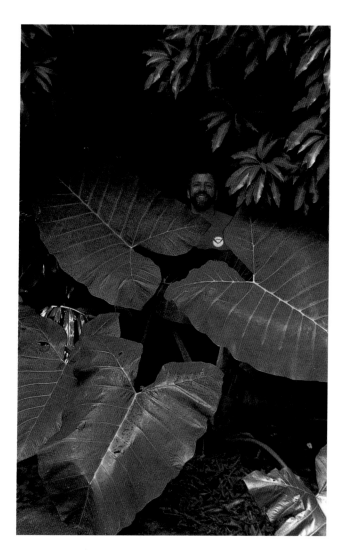

Elephant ears are named for their giant leaves. All parts of these plants contain needlelike calcium oxalate crystals, made harmless by cooking. Ancient Hawaiians, who named this plant 'ape, ate its roots during times of famine. (Susan Scott)

The amount of calcium oxalate in a plant varies greatly from species to species and often even within the same species.

A person must crush or chew the leaf, flower, or stem of these plants to produce symptoms. That kind of mechanical action causes special cells in the plant to inject the needle-sharp calcium oxalate crystals into the skin or mucosa. Chewing or crushing also causes the release of an enzyme that produces redness and swelling.

Brief sucking on, or licking of, a leaf or flower is not usually toxic.

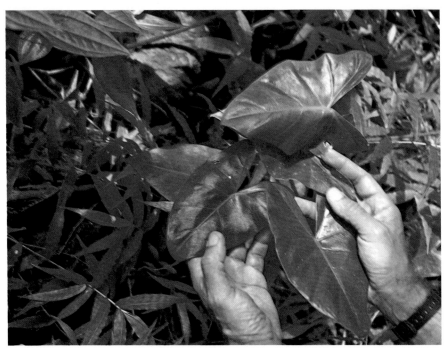

Some elephant ears have relatively small leaves, but the leaves of all types, large and small, contain bundles of calcium oxalate crystals. If the leaves are eaten raw, these crystals can cause pain and swelling in the lips, mouth, and throat. (Susan Scott)

# Traditional and Modern Uses

Ancient Hawaiians wrapped fever victims in 'ape leaves to induce sweating. In ancient Tahiti, people applied juice of this plant to wounds to promote healing. Traditional uses of 'ape like these are scientifically unproven and may be harmful.

Ancient Hawaiians planted 'ape near a gate or fence, believing the irritating sap of the leaves would ward off evil spirits. 'Ape leaves placed under the sleeping mats of the sick, or tied around the body, were for a similar purpose. People did not plant 'ape near the house for fear the inhabitants would become ill.

Ancient Hawaiians used 'ape leaves and stems to make a dye for decorating gourd bowls. 'Ape roots were eaten only as famine food. In Guatemala, elephant ear leaves make good emergency umbrellas, as well as cooked food.

# Incidence

Because elephant ears are low growing, easily accessible, and interesting to play with, these plants frequently injure children. In 1997, the Hawaii Poison Center received calls from ten people exposed to elephant ears; in 1998, six people called. These numbers represent only a fraction of the number of elephant ear exposures experienced by Hawai'i residents and visitors.

In one Florida case, three children chewed on elephant ear stems, believing them to be sugarcane. In another Florida incident, three children ate the stems thinking them celery.

Because stinging in the mouth occurs so quickly, children rarely swallow any of the plant. In Australia, though, at least two deaths have been attributed to the eating of the elephant ear *Alocasia macrorrhizos.* Both victims were children.

Adults sometimes eat elephant ears undercooked. In one Florida case, a woman who boiled the base of an elephant ear plant twice, then tasted a teaspoon of it, had a sore throat for ten days. More than three weeks later, her voice and throat were still abnormal. Because these painful symptoms begin immediately, victims rarely swallow much of the undercooked root.

# Signs and Symptoms

Occasionally, a red, itching rash develops when the juice of one of these plants gets on the skin. Juice in the eye causes immediate pain, tearing, and sensitivity to light.

The main symptom of eating raw or undercooked calcium oxalate crystals is immediate pain followed by swelling of the lips, mouth, tongue, and throat. Some people have described it as pins-and-needles pain. The victim often has excessive salivation, and blisters sometimes develop. Speaking may be difficult or impossible for up to 2 days. Swelling of the throat may cause difficulty breathing.

If a victim swallows any of this uncooked plant, vomiting and diarrhea may follow.

# First Aid

The pain and swelling from calcium oxalate crystals usually disappear slowly without special therapy.

Wash exposed skin immediately with soap and water. Try lifting embedded crystals with sticky tape. If the rash itches persistently, try 1 percent hydrocortisone cream 4 times a day, and 1 or 2 25-milligram diphenhydramine (Benadryl) tablets every 6 hours. Diphenhydramine may cause drowsiness: Do not drive, swim, or surf after taking this medication. Give children diphenhydramine syrup, following the dosage directions on the package.

For juice in the eye, rinse with large amounts of tap water for at least 15 minutes. Go to an emergency room for blurry vision, swelling, or prolonged pain.

If when tasting any part of this plant, even if it is cooked, you feel a burning sensation in your mouth, spit out all of the plant. Immediately rinse your mouth with water and spit that out, too. Try sucking on ice cubes to relieve the pain. Do not swallow the ice water.

If any swelling occurs in the face, mouth, or throat, or if a victim has any difficulty breathing, call 911. Take leaves and stems of the plant to the emergency room for identification.

# Advanced Medical Treatment

No specific antidote or clinically useful diagnostic test exists for calcium oxalate rash, eye exposure, or ingestion. Most cases have only local symptoms that usually respond to first aid treatment.

Calcium oxalate crystals do not dissolve in the digestive tract and therefore do not cause systemic poisoning. They can, however, cause severe burning pain, hematemesis, and bloody diarrhea.

Sap in the eyes may cause corneal abrasions or deposits of calcium oxalate crystals on the cornea. Irrigate thoroughly and examine with a slit lamp. Ocular steroids are unproven but are reasonable to try.

Pain medication may be necessary for both ocular and oral pain.

# FOXGLOVE
## *(Digitalis purpurea)*

Foxglove grows to about 4 feet tall and is a native of Europe. This plant thrives in gardens in cooler regions of North America, including Canada and Alaska. In Hawaiʻi, foxglove grows only at fairly high altitudes.

People grow foxglove for the drooping, bell-shaped flowers, which come in spotted purple, white, and red. These velvety, 3-inch-long flowers are popular in the florist trade.

## Toxin

All parts of the foxglove plant contain digitoxin, a cardiac glycoside. Cardiac glycosides block normal electrical impulses throughout the body, including the heart, by interfering with the exchange of sodium and potassium in and out of nerve and muscle cells.

Juice from this plant contains saponins that can irritate eyes and skin. Inhaling plant dust while raking foxglove leaves may irritate the nose and throat.

People experience a wide range of responses after eating plants containing cardiac glycosides. Some barely become sick; others have died. Regard all parts of this plant, either green or dried, as extremely toxic. Inhaling smoke from burning foxglove plants may cause poisoning.

## Traditional and Modern Uses

For centuries, people have used foxglove leaves to treat heart disease. However, because dosage is inconsistent from leaf to leaf, this practice was and is highly dangerous. Folk remedies using foxglove can easily result in death.

Today, physicians almost exclusively use a similar drug, digoxin, a cardiac glycoside derived from a close relative of foxglove, *Digitalis lanata*. However, even though dosage is precise, digoxin still has a narrow safety range and a high incidence of toxicity.

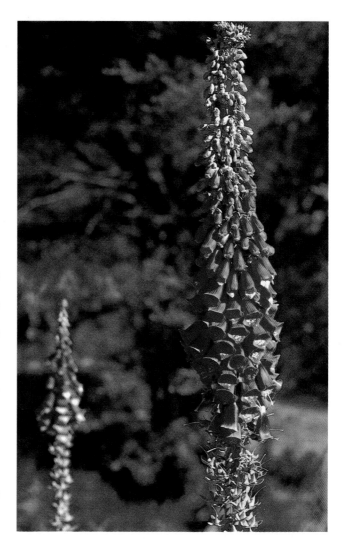

Foxglove grows best in cool climates and is not common in Hawai'i. It does grow in some up-slope gardens, though, and occasionally appears in florists' bouquets. Foxglove contains the powerful heart drug digitoxin. *(Keith Leber)*

## Incidence

Foxglove poisoning is rare in Hawai'i. The plants do not grow wild here, and the cultivated ones grow only at high altitudes.

In 1997, the Hawaii Poison Center received one call from a person with foxglove exposure; in 1998, there were no calls.

## Signs and Symptoms

Skin contact with foxglove leaves can cause a red, itching rash. Sap in the eyes can cause tearing and redness.

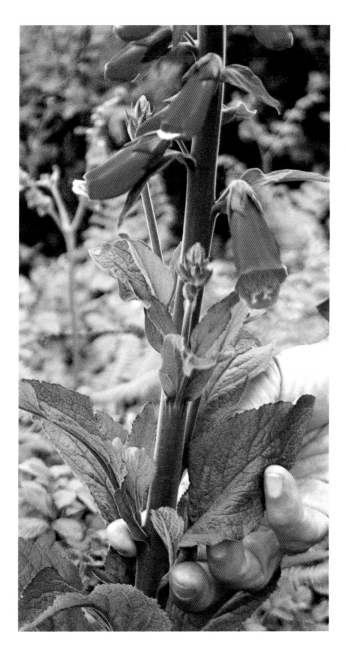

Though all parts of the foxglove plant contain digitoxin, healers in the past used mainly the plant's leaves to treat heart disease. Because of the difficulty of measuring dosage in a particular leaf, this practice was, and is, extremely dangerous, sometimes resulting in death. *(Susan Scott)*

People who eat any part of a foxglove plant may have immediate burning, redness, and swelling of the lips and mouth.

Swallowing this plant can cause the victim to have nausea, vomiting, abdominal pain, and cramping. This can go on for several hours before the generalized heart symptoms begin, including slow or irregular heartbeat, dizziness, headache, and confusion. Victims may feel drowsy or giddy.

## First Aid

Thoroughly wash skin exposed to foxglove sap with soap and water. Rinse exposed eyes for at least 15 minutes with tap water. For persistent itching or blurred vision, consult a doctor.

Regard the swallowing of any part of this plant as a medical emergency. Call 911. Take the entire plant to the emergency room for identification.

## Advanced Medical Treatment

Foxglove plants contain several cardiac glycocides, including digitoxin. Therefore, laboratory blood tests for digoxin or digitoxin may be positive for some foxglove poisonings. Because these tests rely on cross-reactivity between the plant's cardiac glycosides and digoxin or digitoxin, serum levels do not necessarily correlate with biological activity. A low digoxin or digitoxin level may indicate a potentially fatal level of foxglove cardiac glycosides.

An elevated potassium level in the presence of a plant inges-tion suggests cardiac glycoside exposure.

If the patient has swallowed foxglove an hour or less before going to the ER, empty the stomach. For all patients suspected of eating foxglove, regardless of time elapsed, give charcoal.

Victims suspected of eating plants containing cardiac glyco-sides require cardiac monitoring. However, the effect of cardiac glycosides on the heart may be delayed; monitor asymptomatic patients for at least 12 hours before discharge.

For life-threatening arrythmias, hyperkalemia, prolonged PR intervals, widened QRS segments, or altered mental status, administer 10 vials of digoxin immune FAB intravenously. In one case of cardiac glycoside poisoning from oleander, the patient woke up 4 minutes after FAB treatment was begun, and his potassium level normalized in 1 hour. If improvement is minimal, give another 10 vials. The cross-reactivity for binding may require a high concentration of digoxin immune FAB.

The risks of digoxin immune FAB include fever, apnea, hypokalemia, and hypoglycemia. Rebound toxicity occurs in

3 to 11 days in a small fraction of patients treated with digoxin immune FAB. Some researchers suggest a continuous FAB infusion after an initial bolus. Hemoperfusion and forced diuresis are of no benefit.

If FAB is unavailable, use IV atropine to treat bradycardia, and use lidocaine, amiodarone, or phenytoin for ventricular arrythmias. Consider phenytoin or a pacemaker in victims with second- or third-degree heart block.

# GLORIOSA LILY
## (Gloriosa superba)

The gloriosa lily is a flowering vine from tropical Asia and tropical and subtropical Africa. The vine is notable for its exquisitely beautiful 3-inch flowers. The leaves curl at the tip, forming tendrils that enable the plant to climb 10 feet or higher.

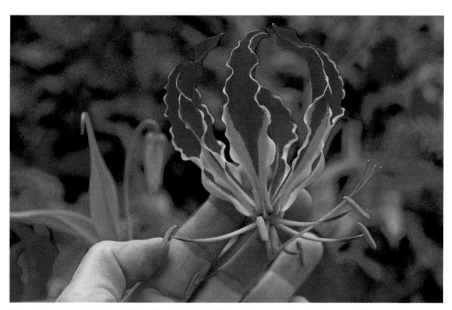

People grow gloriosa lilies for their striking flowers, but the yamlike roots sometimes cause trouble. Though all of the plant contains toxin, it is most concentrated in the root. Just a tiny portion of the root can kill an adult. *(Susan Scott)*

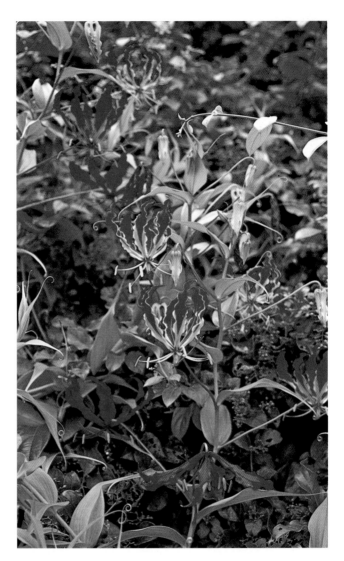

At their peak, the petals of gloriosa lily blossoms are red and yellow and turn up (center flowers). The petals of older flowers turn solid red, then bend down (bottom flowers). *(Craig Thomas)*

*Gloriosa superba* flowers are bright red and yellow, with petals curled back and six projecting stamens. After the flowers bloom, the plants form 3-inch-long seedpods and die back. Underground, the plant grows a tuberous root about a foot long and more than an inch wide. People who mistake this root for a yam or sweet potato make a regrettable error, for it is highly poisonous.

# Toxin

All parts of gloriosa lilies contain colchicine, an alkaloid-like toxin. Colchicine's mechanism of action is not completely understood, but its toxicity may have to do with its ability to stop cell division.

The roots of gloriosa lilies are particularly toxic. Less than one-tenth ounce of gloriosa root contains a potentially fatal dose of colchicine.

# Traditional and Modern Uses

Colchicine is a prescription medication used to treat gout. Molecular biologists also use colchicine in research because it stops cell division while still allowing chromosome duplication.

In India and Burma, people have used gloriosa root to kill themselves and to kill others. In Africa and Asia, people have used the juice from these plants as folk medicine, sometimes with fatal results. The use of any part of a gloriosa lily as a remedy is scientifically unproven and extremely dangerous; it may even cause death. Three drops of gloriosa juice has killed a dog.

# Incidence

Gloriosa plant poisoning is rare in Hawai'i. In 1997 and 1998, the Hawaii Poison Center received no calls from people with gloriosa exposure. However, at least six people worldwide have died from eating gloriosa root. Death occurred from one to eight days after eating.

A woman in Sri Lanka became seriously ill after eating a gloriosa root she mistook for a yam. She recovered.

# Signs and Symptoms

Eating any part of a gloriosa lily can cause numbness of the lips, tongue, and throat. Some people feel a burning sensation in the mouth and throat.

From 2 to 12 hours may pass without any more symptoms. Later, nausea, vomiting, diarrhea (sometimes bloody), abdominal pain, chest pain, and rapid heartbeat are common symptoms. In severe cases, the symptoms progress to slow heart beat, seizures, confusion, coma, and possibly paralysis 24 to 72 hours after eating the plant. Occasionally, the victim has a fever or blurred vision.

Death from cardiac or respiratory failure can occur within 7 hours.

## First Aid

Regard as a medical emergency the eating of any part of any gloriosa lily, even if the victim shows no symptoms. Go directly to the nearest emergency room. If symptoms have begun, or if the victim has any difficulty breathing, call 911. Take flowers, leaves, and roots of the plant to the emergency room for identification.

## Advanced Medical Treatment

No antidote or diagnostic test exists for colchicine poisoning. Obtain laboratory screening tests, including baseline liver and renal function tests.

Colchicine poisoning occurs in three phases. The first is gastrointestinal, occurring 2 to 12 hours after ingestion. Give charcoal; replace fluids and electrolytes as necessary.

The second phase is multisystem failure, occurring in 24 to 72 hours and characterized by fever, ascending neuropathy, and cardiovascular toxicity. Direct treatment at life support. Be prepared to protect the airway. Death occurs from respiratory failure, cardiovascular collapse, asystole, or sepsis 3 to 7 days later.

If the patient survives, the third phase is recovery, occurring 7 to 10 days after ingestion. Fever may persist for several weeks. The patient often experiences rebound leukocytosis and reversible hair loss.

Because colchicine is widely distributed throughout the body, hemodialysis is of no benefit in colchicine poisoning.

# HAWAIIAN POPPY
## (Argemone glauca)

The Hawaiian poppy, or *pua kala*, is Hawai'i's only native poppy. Captain Cook's surgeon and botanist William Anderson collected one from Waimea, Kaua'i, during Cook's third voyage, in 1778.

The *pua kala* belongs to the poppy family and is related to the opium poppy, *Papaver somniferum*. About two hundred species of the poppy family grow throughout the world.

The Hawaiian poppy grows 2 to 5 feet tall and bears white flowers similar to other poppies. Prickles cover *pua kala* leaves and seedpods, and a thin, waxy coating covers the entire plant, thus slowing evaporation. Because of this, Hawaiian poppies grow well in dry, rocky areas from sea level to about 9,000 feet.

Few of Hawai'i's native plants are poisonous. The Hawaiian poppy, however, is one of these unusual plants. This species is now uncommon, growing only on a few dry, leeward coasts.

A close relative of the Hawaiian poppy is the Mexican poppy *(Argemone mexicana)*, cultivated in Hawai'i at least since 1934 and now naturalized. The Mexican poppy bears yellow flowers in Hawai'i and grows wild in dry, disturbed areas. It, too, is poisonous.

## Toxin

The Hawaiian poppy contains a thick, yellow juice in the stems, leaves, and roots; all parts bearing this sap are toxic. The toxins in the juice are unknown alkaloids, probably similar to those in Mexican poppies and another relative, *Argemone alba*, a poppy common in India. The alkaloids irritate the stomach and intestines.

*Pua kala* extract administered to mice resulted in respiratory depression and deep sleep. Higher concentrations caused seizures and death.

## Traditional and Modern Uses

Ancient Hawaiians used *pua kala* for toothache, pounding and heating the rind, then placing it on the sore tooth. They also

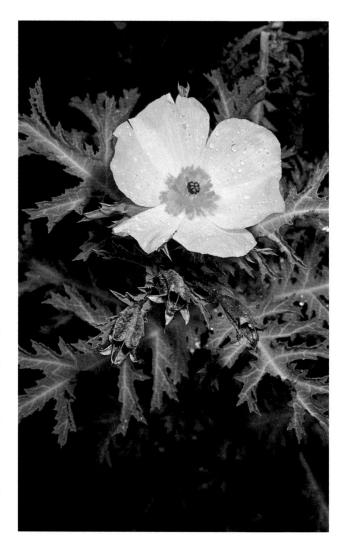

The Hawaiian poppy is one of the few Hawaiian native plants toxic to humans. The poison is in the thick yellow sap that runs through the stems, leaves, and roots of this prickly plant. *(Art Whistler)*

applied the juice to warts, letting it dry in the sun. This was repeated until the wart fell off. Healers applied *pua kala* on open wounds to aid healing.

Using the Hawaiian poppy as a remedy is scientifically unproven and may be harmful.

# Incidence

The sap of the Hawaiian poppy is extremely bitter. This, along with the scarcity of the plant, makes poisonings extremely rare.

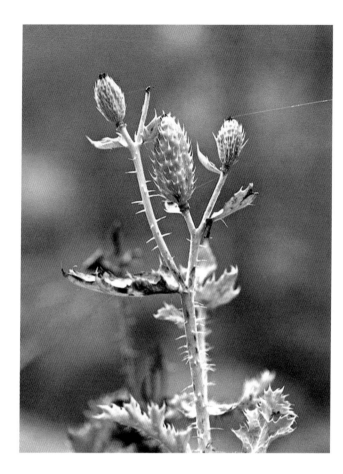

Most Hawaiian poppies, or *pua kala,* have prickles covering their leaves, stems, and seedpods. *(Susan Scott)*

Even livestock shun the plant because of its prickly exterior and bitter taste. In 1997 and 1998, the Hawaii Poison Center received no calls from people with Hawaiian poppy exposure.

People have been poisoned in India from the Indian poppy, *Argemone alba*, when the plant was accidentally mixed in with homegrown wheat, oats, and corn.

## Signs and Symptoms

Because no specific cases of Hawaiian poppy poisoning have been published, precise symptoms are unknown. The symptoms probably resemble those of Mexican poppy ingestion: vomiting, diarrhea, visual disturbances, swelling of the abdomen, fainting, and coma. An irregular heartbeat is a possibility, because the toxin can affect the heart muscles.

Based on experiments with mice, victims may experience slowed breathing, a deep sleep, seizures, and death.

## First Aid

Because little is known about this toxin, it is wise to regard it as potentially lethal. Poisoning victims should go to an emergency room. If symptoms are severe, or the victim has any difficulty breathing, call 911. Take the entire plant to the emergency room for identification.

## Advanced Medical Treatment

The alkaloid in this plant is unknown; no antidote or diagnostic test exists for poisoning from it. The related Mexican poppy contains multiple toxic alkaloids, with gastrointestinal, cardiac, and central nervous system effects.

Give charcoal; replace fluids and electrolytes as needed. Direct treatment at life support and relieving symptoms.

# HYDRANGEA
## *(Hydrangea macrophylla)*

Hydrangeas are natives of eastern Asia. In Hawai'i, they grow as shrubs, particularly at high, cool altitudes.

People raise hydrangeas for their large bundles of blue, pink, or white flowers. The bushes grow 3 to 12 feet tall.

Flower colors of hydrangeas vary with soil nutrients. Untreated Hawai'i soil produces blue or white flowers; adding lime to the soil produces pink flowers.

## Toxin

All parts of the hydrangea contain hydrangin, a cyanogenic glycoside that breaks down to cyanide when eaten. This chemical process takes place slowly in an acid environment, as in the stomach, but takes place rapidly in an alkaline environment, as in the small intestine.

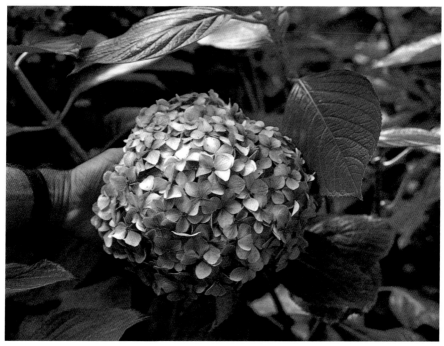

All parts of the hydrangea plant contain a potentially lethal poison, which can turn to cyanide in the human body. When the authors spotted hydrangea flowers around the edges of a buffet salad at a local bed and breakfast establishment, they alerted the proprietor. "Oh, that's just for decoration," she replied. "You aren't supposed to eat it." Perhaps disbelieving the potential danger, she left the flowers in the salad. *(Susan Scott)*

Cyanide is extremely toxic to humans because it makes the body's cells unable to use oxygen.

## Traditional and Modern Uses

People in Japan use steamed hydrangea leaves in a drink. This practice is dangerous and could possibly result in death.

## Incidence

Accidental poisonings from hydrangea are rare. In 1997 and 1998, the Hawaii Poison Center received no calls from people with hydrangea exposure.

When poisonings do occur, people invariably have used hydrangea plant parts as food, such as putting hydrangea flower

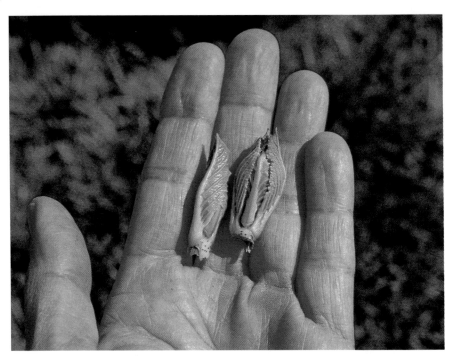

People have been poisoned after eating hydrangea flower buds, such as these, in salads. Today, when edible flowers in salads are becoming increasingly popular, it pays to know which plants are safe to eat and which are potentially dangerous. *(Susan Scott)*

buds in salads. In the few reported cases of hydrangea poisonings, the symptoms were those of stomach upset rather than cyanide poisoning.

## Signs and Symptoms

Eating hydrangea buds usually causes sudden, severe vomiting and stomach pain. If any of the plant remains in the stomach or intestine, overall cyanide poisoning is possible.

Because the chemical reaction that produces cyanide is delayed in the stomach by the acid there, symptoms of cyanide poisoning may take 1/2 to 2 hours or longer after swallowing this plant. Once the cyanide is formed, the victim at first feels dizzy and tired. Mucus membranes, nail beds, and skin may be bluish, but this sign is not always present in cyanide poisoning.

In severe poisonings, victims may suffer rapid, then slowed breathing, seizures, muscle weakness, loss of bladder control, and coma.

## First Aid

Because hydrangeas are capable of producing cyanide, regard the eating of any of it as a medical emergency. Go directly to the nearest emergency room. If symptoms have already begun, or if the victim has any difficulty breathing, call 911. Take flowers, stems, and buds of the plant to the emergency room for identification.

## Advanced Medical Treatment

If the patient is symptomatic, give charcoal. Victims require cardiac monitoring and 100 percent oxygen therapy.

For patients with significant symptoms, such as loss of consciousness, unstable vital signs, seizures, or acidosis, use the cyanide antidote kit.

Obtain baseline arterial blood gases, electrolytes, lactate, and cyanide levels. Do not delay therapy for results of cyanide testing. Monitor methemoglobin levels in patients receiving treatment from the kit. Dialysis after the kit treatment may improve acidosis and remove thiocyanate from the blood.

Chronic poisoning occurs in people eating cyanogenic diets and causes neuropathy with color blindness, deafness, spastic paraparesis, and ataxia. The seeds and pits of apples, apricots, cherries, peaches, plums, as well as lima beans, sorghum, and cassava contain cyanogenic glycosides. The crushed seeds of some of these are sold as "health foods," vitamin supplements, or cancer remedies.

# JAPANESE ANEMONE
## (Anemone hupehensis)

The Japanese anemone is native to Japan and China. People in Hawai'i grow them for their showy white, pink, red, or purple flowers, which bloom in the fall.

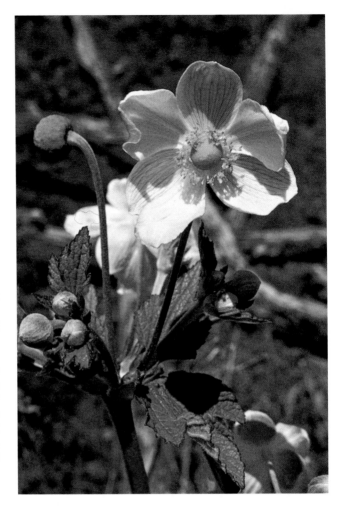

All parts of Japanese anemones contain a toxin that can cause blisters on the skin and mucus membranes. The toxin is most concentrated when the plant is flowering. After flowering, the green sphere at the flower's center (pictured) breaks open and releases seeds. *(Art Whistler)*

Japanese anemones grow to about 3 feet tall and do well in cool regions of the Islands. The plants grow wild in wet, disturbed areas, such as roadsides in and around Hawai'i Volcanoes National Park on the island of Hawai'i.

## Toxin

All parts of the Japanese anemone contain ranunculin, a glucoside that hydrolyzes to protoanemonin. This toxin can cause blisters on skin and mucus membranes. Because the juice of this plant tastes exceedingly bitter, generalized poisonings are extremely rare.

The amount of toxin in each anemone varies widely. The toxin is most concentrated while the plant is flowering. Heat or drying destroys protoanemonin.

## Traditional and Modern Uses

Medical researchers have studied protoanemonin for its antibiotic properties. It may also be useful in the treatment of leukemia.

Using any part of the Japanese anemone as a remedy is scientifically unproven and may be harmful.

## Incidence

Japanese anemone poisoning is rare. In 1997 and 1998, the Hawaii Poison Center received no calls from people with Japanese anemone exposure.

The taste of this plant is so bad and painful to the mouth,

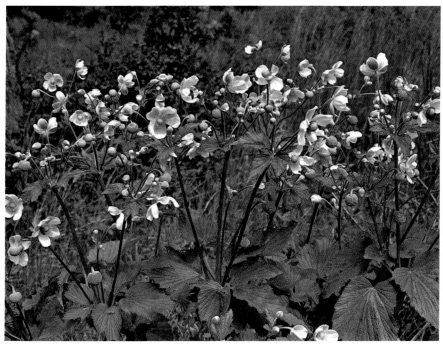

Japanese anemones grow wild in parts of Volcanoes National Park on the island of Hawai'i. This stand is 3 to 4 feet tall. *(Susan Scott)*

most people spit it out immediately. If swallowed, the toxin causes intense vomiting, thereby usually eliminating itself from the body.

# Signs and Symptoms

Anemone juice in the eye can cause redness, pain, swelling, tearing, sensitivity to light, and possible blurred vision. On the skin, anemone juice can cause itching, burning, redness, swelling, and blisters. Sometimes, the skin darkens at the contact area.

Eating any part of this plant causes an immediate burning sensation and possibly blisters in the mouth and throat. Saliva production may increase greatly.

If swallowed, the toxin causes stomach pain, vomiting, and diarrhea, possibly bloody. Dizziness sometimes follows, with possible seizures and/or kidney damage.

 ## First Aid

Rinse eyes exposed to Japanese anemone with large amounts of tap water for 15 minutes. Wash exposed skin thoroughly with soap and water. If symptoms persist or become unbearable, contact a doctor.

If you suspect that a child has eaten any part of a Japanese anemone, take them to the nearest emergency room. If symptoms are severe, such as vomiting blood, or the victim has any difficulty breathing, call 911. Take flowers, stems, and leaves of the plant to the emergency room for identification.

 ## Advanced Medical Treatment

No specific antidote or diagnostic test exists for Japanese anemone poisoning. Decontaminate exposure areas. Blistering with subsequent hyperpigmentation can occur after skin exposure. Treat the area as a burn. Instruct the patient to use sunscreen to minimize the risk of hyperpigmentation.

Systemic poisonings are extremely rare because of immediate, intense vomiting after swallowing this plant. Direct treatment at controlling emesis. Give charcoal; replace fluids and electrolytes as needed. Be prepared to treat seizures.

Neurologic and genitourinary problems have occurred in poisoned animals. Serious exposures in humans are rare. Visual impairment sometimes occurs in animals grazing on this plant.

# JATROPHA
## (*Jatropha* species)

Jatropha plants are a diverse group, having up to 175 species. Most are native to tropical America but now are cultivated widely throughout the world.

People grow jatropha plants as hedges, shrubs, and for their bright flowers. One of these is the coral plant (*J. multifida*), named for its red flowers, which cluster together like certain kinds of coral.

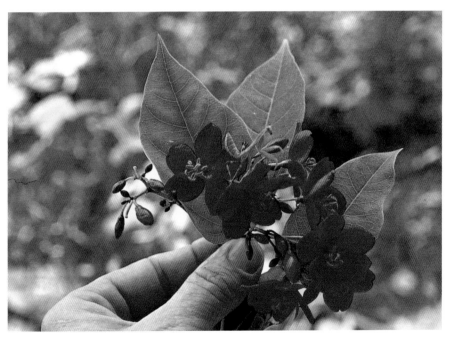

This rose-flowered jatropha (adorned with a young praying mantis) is a popular ornamental shrub in Hawai'i. All jatropha plants contain various amounts of curcin, a dangerous toxin. Regard all parts of all jatropha plants as potentially lethal. *(Susan Scott)*

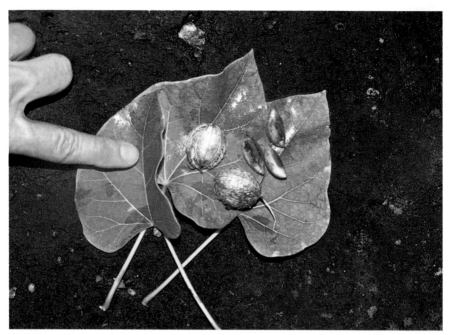

These *Jatropha curcas* nuts are called physic nuts. Each nut consists of three seeds, shown. Oil from the nuts is nicknamed "hell oil" after its potent action as a laxative. The poison curcin is particularly strong in the seeds of these and other jatropha plants. *(Susan Scott)*

The rose-flowered jatropha *(J. integerrima)* is another popular flower in Hawai'i. This bush produces red flowers about 1 inch across, also in clusters.

Other jatrophas in Hawai'i are the cotton-leafed jatropha *(J. gossypiifolia)*, the physic nut, or *kuku'ihi (J. curcas)*, and the gout plant *(J. podagrica)*.

The roundish fruits of jatropha plants range from one-half to one and one-half inches long; they are first green, then turn brown. Each contains three tasty but potentially lethal, poisonous seeds. The leaves and milky sap of all these plants also are poisonous.

## Toxin

Jatropha plants contain a potentially lethal toxin, curcin, which is a type of toxalbumin. Toxalbumins cause bleeding lesions in the mouth, esophagus, stomach, and intestines. The lesions resemble alkaline burns, though the onset is sometimes delayed several hours after ingestion. Once absorbed into the bloodstream, toxalbumins interfere with cell function and cause cell damage, leading to serious liver, kidney, adrenal, and nerve damage and sometimes death.

The entire jatropha plant is toxic, but by far the most potent part is the seeds. The toxicity of the seeds, however, is variable. Some may be lethal; others may be nontoxic. Toxicity varies even within the same species. The degree of poisoning a person experiences may depend on how thoroughly the victim chewed the seeds.

Though not closely related scientifically to jatropha plants, black-eyed Susan seeds and castor beans also contain toxalbumins.

Jatropha plants also contain saponins, glycosides that are surface-active substances with detergent-like properties.

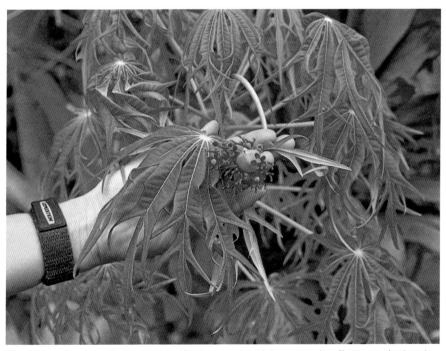

This jatropha is called a coral plant, so-named because its flowers cluster together like some corals. All parts of jatropha plants are poisonous, but the seeds (the green, four-sided sphere among the red flowers) are the most potent. (Susan Scott)

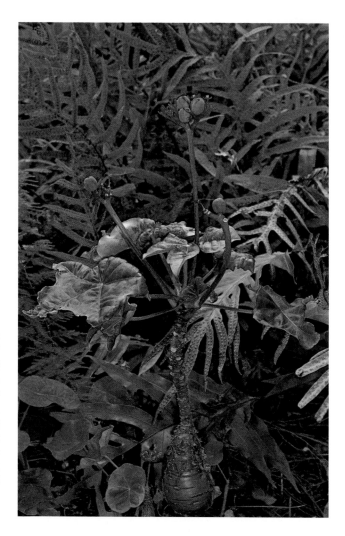

The gout plant is another type of jatropha. This species is easy to identify by its swollen base. Flowers and seeds of the gout plant are similar to those of the coral plant. *(Susan Scott)*

# Traditional and Modern Uses

Oil from the physic nut plant, or *kukuʻihi*, is extremely potent; the oil's nickname is hell oil. People once commonly used this oil as a laxative but discontinued the practice because of its potential toxicity. Despite the danger, however, people in some tropical countries still use the oil as a folk remedy for various ailments. The sap of the physic nut plant is sometimes used to stop a cut from bleeding. In the Philippines, people use the leaves for treating snake bite, insect stings, boils, toothache, scabies, eczema, rheumatism, and ringworm.

Today, physic nut oil is used in soaps and candles. In Africa, people grind up physic nuts and mix them with palm oil for use as rat poison.

Philippines fishermen use the leaves of the cotton-leafed jatropha to poison fish. In Aruba, people believe the peeled and mashed stem of this plant cures throat cancer. Costa Ricans attribute the cotton-leafed jatropha with being a cancer cure, a belief that may have some validity. U.S. researchers have found some antitumor properties in the roots of this species.

Using any part of a jatropha plant as a remedy is scientifically unproven. It may be harmful or even cause death.

# Incidence

Jatropha poisonings are rare. In 1997 and 1998, Hawaii Poison Center received no calls from people with jatropha exposure. In the past, however, children in Hawai'i have been poisoned by eating the sweet seeds of jatropha. None of these cases were fatal.

Toxicity varies widely in jatropha plants, even within the same species. People have become violently ill after eating only one physic nut seed. In another case, a person who ate fifty seeds experienced only mild symptoms.

Three deaths have been reported in Africa from eating coral plant seeds.

# Signs and Symptoms

In the eyes, sap from jatropha leaves and stems can cause redness, tearing, and swelling. Eating physic nuts may cause either dilated or constricted pupils.

Occasionally, the sap of some of these plants on the skin causes a rash.

A person who has swallowed jatropha seeds can develop symptoms anywhere from 6 hours to 3 days later. Then, the victim may have a burning sensation in the mouth and throat, followed by nausea, vomiting, and diarrhea, often with bleeding.

In severe cases, open sores form in the mouth, esophagus, and throughout the stomach and intestines. These symptoms resemble chemical burns. Blood in the urine is common. Dehydration follows, then death as a result of fluid loss or, later, organ failure.

In one study of jatropha ingestions in the Philippines, 64 percent of victims developed vomiting, 52 percent had abdominal pain, and 98 percent were discharged from the hospital 24 to 48 hours after poisoning.

# First Aid

Wash intact, exposed skin thoroughly with soap and water. See a physician if the skin continues to be irritated and painful.

Because the toxin of jatropha plants is potentially fatal, getting any part of these plants in a cut, in the eyes, or in the body by swallowing should be regarded as a medical emergency. Call 911. Take the seeds, and the rest of the plant if available, to the emergency department for identification.

# Advanced Medical Treatment

No specific antidote or clinically useful diagnostic test exists for toxalbumin poisoning. Make the diagnosis by physical exam and history. Either absorbed through a cut or eaten, this toxin is life-threatening because of potential shock from fluid and electrolyte loss.

Decontaminate exposed skin and eyes. Examine eyes with a slit lamp and perform funduscopic exam to check for both pupillary dilation and constriction. Retinal hemorrhage and optic neuritis have been reported.

Gastrointestinal injury is similar to caustic alkaline burns, though the onset is delayed 2 to 3 hours after ingestion.

Keep asymptomatic patients who are suspected of swallowing one or more seeds under observation for at least 8 hours. Instruct care-givers to call 911 immediately if symptoms begin later at home.

For ingestions, give charcoal. Be prepared to treat for shock. Late complications occur after a 2 to 5–day asymptomatic period and are caused by toxic injury to liver, kidney, adrenal, and central nervous system damage.

Even with intensive care, the ingestion of one seed can be fatal. Conversely, people who have eaten numerous seeds have experienced no illness.

# JIMSONWEED
## (Datura stramonium)

Jimsonweed, or thorn apple, is native to the southern United States. The plant has been growing wild in Hawai'i at least since 1871. Today, this foul-smelling plant, with trumpet-shaped flowers and prickly seedpods, is an occasional weed in dry, disturbed areas, such as pastures and roadsides.

The term *jimson* is a corruption of the name Jamestown, the early English colony in Virginia. In 1676, British soldiers sent there to suppress Bacon's Rebellion ate leaves of this plant and became ill for several days. The plant was named Jamestown weed, or jimsonweed.

Hawaiian names for this weed are *kīkānia haole* and *lā'au hānō*.

A close relative of jimsonweed is the garden *Datura (D. metel)*, also known as cornucopia or horn-of-plenty. These plants, native to Central America, were transported to Hawai'i around 1900. Today, they occasionally grow in gardens and in the wild.

Jimsonweed and other *Datura* species are closely related to angel's trumpets and have the same toxins.

## Toxin

The entire jimsonweed plant is toxic, containing the alkaloids atropine, hyoscyamine, and scopolamine. These chemicals affect the central nervous system.

Many jimsonweed poisonings are the result of people trying to induce a hallucinogenic high. Often, overdoses occur in adolescents who do not realize the potency of the drug.

The toxicity of jimsonweed varies year by year and from plant to plant. It even varies among leaves of the same plant. The seeds have the highest concentrations of toxins.

## Traditional and Modern Uses

American Indians traditionally have used jimsonweed for medicine and in religious ceremonies. Aztecs have used a *Datura* species as a magic, vision-producing drug.

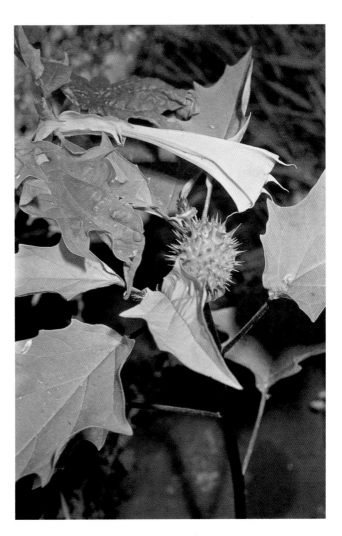

Jimsonweed (also called thorn apple), a close relative of angel's trumpet, is highly poisonous. Most jimsonweed poisonings are intentional, a result of the victims trying to get high. The weed has caused death when combined with alcohol. *(Art Whistler)*

People practicing traditional Chinese medicine use *Datura* plants to treat asthma, bronchitis, pain, seizures, psychosis, and the flu. In some parts of Brazil, people apply extracts and pastes made of jimsonweed and its relatives to the skin to treat inflammation and injuries. Such traditional uses of this plant are scientifically unproven; some may be harmful.

Several *Datura* species are grown in the United States, Europe, and Asia for use in pharmaceuticals.

People in Iran use *Datura* seeds to kill dogs, and in Africa, the seeds are used as insecticides.

Criminals have been known to mix *Datura metel* seeds in a drink, or have blown powered seeds into someone's bedroom at night, to stupefy and then rob the victim. Murderers have mixed the seeds in food, thus killing their victims.

# Incidence

Jimsonweed is the most commonly abused plant requiring medical care in the United States. In Hawai'i, however, abuse is apparently less common than on the mainland. In 1997, the Hawaii Poison Center received calls from two people exposed to jimsonweed; in 1998, there were no calls.

In 1993, the American Association of Poison Control Centers Toxic Surveillance System received 318 reports of jimsonweed exposure. In 1994, four teen-age boys in Texas drank tea made from jimsonweed roots and alcohol. Two of them died.

Other serious poisonings in 1994 were in adolescents in New York and California. Some required admission to intensive care units; others were discharged from emergency rooms without treatment. All survived.

One poison center reported an ingestion range of thirty to fifty seeds per person in fourteen cases. The average age was 16.8 years old. All lived.

Several people in Hong Kong became ill after taking the traditional Chinese medicine *ling-xiao-hua*. Researchers later determined that the medicine mistakenly contained *Datura metel* flowers, a close relative of jimsonweed. People in China have become ill after eating ginseng contaminated with *Datura* species.

One Brazilian woman became ill after making and using a toothpaste from a *Datura* plant to treat inflammation of her gums. She did not swallow the substance.

Two adolescents in Belgium were hospitalized with acute psychosis after drinking thorn apple (jimsonweed) tea. Both recovered.

# Signs and Symptoms

Rubbing one or both eyes after handling this plant may cause the pupil(s) to dilate. This results in sensitivity to bright light and blurred vision that can last for about a week.

Symptoms of jimsonweed poisoning usually occur within 30 to 60 minutes after eating and may last for 24 to 48 hours.

Initial symptoms of mild to moderate poisoning include warm skin, dilated pupils (causing blurred vision, and sensitivity to bright light), dry mouth (causing difficulty swallowing and speaking), reddening of the face, restlessness, irritability, disorientation, hallucinations, and/or delirium.

Blurred vision and dilated pupils from eating *Datura* plants may last for 7 to 12 days.

In severe poisonings, victims may feel cold, may be agitated and combative, may be unable to urinate, may have seizures, paralysis, coma, respiratory failure, circulation collapse, and die.

To remember the varied signs and symptoms of this class of drug intoxication, medical doctors traditionally memorize the following phrase: "Hot as a hare, blind as a bat, dry as a bone, red as a beet, and mad as a hatter." The primary characteristic that necessitates admission to the hospital is agitation, so severe it often requires physical restraints.

# First Aid

Wash your hands thoroughly after handling jimsonweed flowers or leaves. Rinse exposed eyes with copious amounts of tap water. If blurred vision persists, consult a doctor.

Mild to moderate cases of jimsonweed poisoning disappear overnight without treatment. For severe symptoms, take the victim to an emergency room. If the victim has any difficulty breathing, call 911. Take as much of the plant as possible to the emergency room for identification.

# Advanced Medical Treatment

No clinically useful diagnostic tests exist for jimsonweed poisoning. Make the diagnosis by physical exam and history. Jimsonweed poisoning presents as atropine poisoning.

Scopolamine and atropine impair peristalsis. Therefore, in severe poisonings, consider emptying the stomach even if more than an hour has elapsed since ingestion. For all ingestions, give charcoal. Catheterize for urinary retention. Use diazepam as necessary for sedation.

Consider physostigmine only for uncontrollable hyperthermia, supraventricular tachycardia with hemodynamic instability, therapy-resistant seizures, and extreme delirium. The recommended dose of physostigmine in adults is 1 to 2 milligrams intravenously over 5 minutes. Repeat every 15 minutes as needed. Never exceed 4 mg in 30 minutes.[1]

For children, start with 0.02 milligrams per kilogram, increasing the dose as necessary to 0.5 mg. Repeat as needed to control symptoms. Maximum dose is 2 mg.[2]

Physostigmine dramatically reverses coma and other anticholinergic symptoms but may itself cause seizures. Never use physostigmine just to keep a patient awake.

# *KĀHILI* FLOWER AND SILKY OAK
## (*Grevillea* species)

*Kāhili* flowers, *Grevillea banksii*, are small trees growing to about 20 feet tall; they are native to Australia. The Hawaiian name *kāhili* comes from the shape of the flower, which resembles the ancient feather staffs of Hawaiian royalty. Another Hawaiian name, *ha'ikū*, comes from the fact that the first trees of this type in Hawai'i grew in Ha'ikū, Maui, around 1900.

*Kāhili* trees were once familiar throughout the Islands, when people grew them for their lovely red or yellow flowers with hairy centers. In the past, these flowers were common in *lei* and bouquets, but because many people are allergic to these flowers, their use is rare today. Though *kāhili* trees are seldom cultivated any more, they grow wild in northeast Kaua'i and in Ka'ū on the island of Hawai'i.

A close relative of *kāhili* flowers, the silky oak (*Grevillea robusta*), also can cause allergic reactions in some people. In Hawai'i, more than 2.2 million silky oaks were planted throughout the main Islands between 1919 and 1959 for timber. These Australia natives grow to 120 feet tall and now grow wild on most Islands. They bloom in spring.

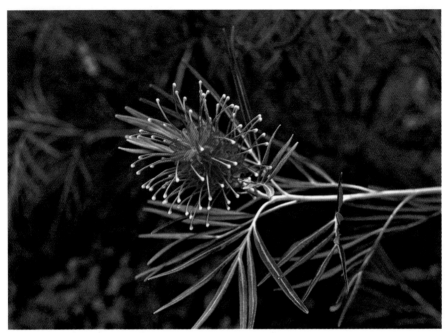

*Kāhili* flowers were once common *lei* flowers, but since so many people develop allergies to them they are no longer common in Hawai'i gardens or in *lei*. *(Charles Lamoureaux)*

## Toxin

The toxins in *kāhili* flowers and silky oaks are related to the toxin in poison ivy. The rash these plants causes resembles poison ivy rash. Also like poison ivy, not everyone is sensitive to it.

Apparently, only the flowers of the *kāhili* plant cause a rash; the leaves, stems, sap, and bark do not. In silky oaks, the entire tree, including sawdust from it, can cause rashes or promote asthma attacks.

Though the rash resembles mango rash, people sensitive to *kāhili* flowers and silky oaks are not necessarily sensitive to mangos, and vice versa.[1]

## Traditional and Modern Uses

If *lei* makers use *kāhili* flowers at all, they use them in hat *lei* rather than head or neck *lei* because of the potential for rash.

These showy flowers are sometimes used in Hawaiʻi floral arrangements.

The beautifully grained wood of silky oaks is popular in Australia for flooring and paneling.

# Incidence

In a 1941 report, a Hawaiʻi dermatologist wrote that the *kāhili* flower had been "by far the most frequent and severe plant sensitizer" in his practice during the previous two years. Today, the *kāhili* flower is not common in Hawaiʻi. In 1997 and 1998, the Hawaii Poison Center received no calls from people reporting *kāhili* flower exposure and only one call from a person with silky oak exposure.

The rash usually appears first on the hands, then shows up later on the face and eyelids. Because the onset of the rash is

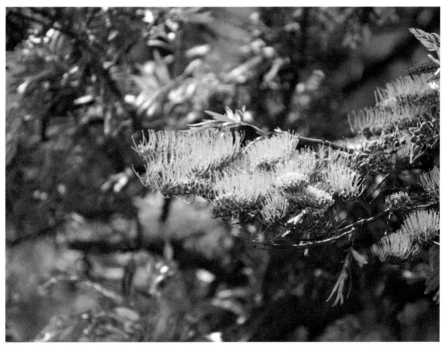

The state of Hawaiʻi planted about 2.2 million silky oak trees between 1919 and 1959 on all the main Islands (except Kahoʻolawe) for lumber. The trees grow to about 100 feet tall and produce orange blossoms in May, June, and July. Some people are allergic to all parts of these trees. (*Craig Thomas*)

usually delayed one to three days after exposure, people rub their faces and eyes without knowing they are spreading the toxin.

In Australia, horses have died after eating parts of these plants. Skin rashes similar to poison ivy are common in India after contact with silky oak trees. In Western Australia, people who are susceptible have asthma attacks when near these trees, and the attacks occur year-round.

## Signs and Symptoms

A severely itchy rash usually occurs 1 to 3 days after exposure. At first, the rash looks like patches of reddened skin. Within 24 hours, tiny blisters form in the red areas, either singly, in narrow lines, or in small clusters. The rash reaches its peak around the sixth day, then gradually disappears over a week or two, leaving no marks.

Being near or in contact with silky oak trees can cause wheezing and difficulty breathing.

 ## First Aid

Wash exposed skin thoroughly with soap and water. For itching, try 1 percent hydrocortisone cream 4 times a day, and 1 or 2 25-milligram diphenhydramine (Benadryl) tablets every 6 hours. Diphenhydramine may cause drowsiness: Do not drive, swim, or surf after taking this medication. Give children diphenhydramine syrup, following the dosage directions on the package.

Consult your doctor about asthma attacks.

If a persistent rash develops, consult a doctor. For facial swelling, any difficulty breathing, or collapse, call 911. Take the *lei* or flowers and leaves with you to the emergency room for identification.

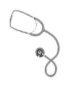 ## Advanced Medical Treatment

No specific antidote or diagnostic test exists for *kāhili* flower or silky oak dermatitis or asthma. Direct treatment at relieving itching, bronchospasm, and other allergy symptoms. For significant rashes, give oral steroids.

# KAVA
## (Piper methysticum)

Kava is a member of the pepper family; its scientific name means intoxicating pepper. This shrub probably originated in Vanuatu. It grows 4 to 12 feet tall, produces heart-shaped leaves, and does not bear fruit in Hawai'i.

Ancient mariners spread kava widely throughout the Pacific islands, including Hawai'i, where it is known as 'awa (pronounced *ah*-vah). More than fifteen varieties were known by ancient Hawaiians, who used it as medicine and tranquilizer. About two hundred varieties of kava are grown throughout the Pacific today, each differing in potency.

In Germany and France, kava is a prescription medicine. In the United States, it can be found in health food stores in the

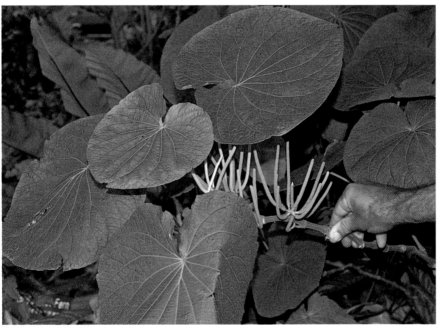

Ancient Polynesian colonists brought kava to Hawai'i, where it grows well. Today, because of its popularity as an alternative medicine for stress and anxiety, people in Hawai'i are growing kava in quantity. Consuming kava can cause stomach pain and/or a skin disorder. *(Susan Scott)*

form of tablets, alcohol tincture, powder, and raw root. Some brand names are Herbal Ecstasy and Kavatrol.

In recent decades, researchers have studied the usefulness of kava in controlling seizures and psychosis. The research was stopped because of the skin disorder that appears with continued use of this drug.

# Toxin

Kava contains about fifteen compounds, kavalactones, that are unique to this plant. Kavalactones depress motor and sensory functions.

Drink made from this plant is nonnarcotic, nonopiate, nonfermented, nonalcoholic, nonhallucinogenic, and physiologically nonaddicting. Drinking kava produces tranquil intoxication, during which thoughts and memory remain clear.

No one knows for sure how kava causes its skin disorder. One theory is that kavalactones may interfere with cholesterol metabolism, thus adversely affecting skin cells that make the fibrous protein keratin. Skin lesions caused by kava are not the result of niacin or tryptophan deficiency (pellagra) or allergy, and are not photoeruptions.

# Traditional and Modern Uses

'Awa was important in ancient Hawaiians' social life, religious ceremonies, and medical treatments.

A drink of 'awa root was made usually for the ali'i (aristocracy) as a pleasure drug; commoners could drink it as a medicine to relax. To make the drink, people chewed 'awa root into a mash, then placed it into a bowl of coconut milk or cold water. To mask the bitter flavor of the drink, 'awa drinkers often ate sweet bananas simultaneously. This accompaniment was called pūpū, which is the origin of the term pūpū for snacks served with drinks.

Some Hawaiian royalty drank 'awa in excess. A member of Captain James Cook's 1778 expedition wrote:

> The Excess with which the Chiefs drink the Kava, destroys their strength & makes them sad objects of Debauchery, they far outdo in the use of this pernicious root all the other Indians we have vist'd; the more Scaly their bodies are, the more honorable it is with them. . . . Many before they are forty are the most miserable

Objects, their whole frame trembles, their Eyes are so sore & redened, they seem in Constant pain; yet I believe in a short time by disusing this liquor the soreness of the eyes goes away; at least we made some of our friends refrain & they recovered amazingly.[1]

As medicine, an '*awa* drink helped sick people sleep, settled down restless children, eased sore muscles after hard work, and relieved the pain of urinary tract infections. '*Awa* was also used to treat asthma and obesity. Packed into the vagina of a pregnant woman, '*awa* leaves were believed to cause an abortion; eating them could cause a miscarriage.

In Samoa, kava (called '*ava* there), is given as medicine for stomachache, backache, and urinary tract infections. Tongans rub the leaves onto centipede bites, insect stings, and fish stings. In the 1850s, Germans imported kava from the Pacific to treat gonorrhea and urinary tract infections. The success of those treatments is unknown.

No controlled studies exist on kava use as an antidepressant.[2] Three controlled German studies, however, suggest kava is an effective alternative treatment for anxiety disorders.[3] The U.S.

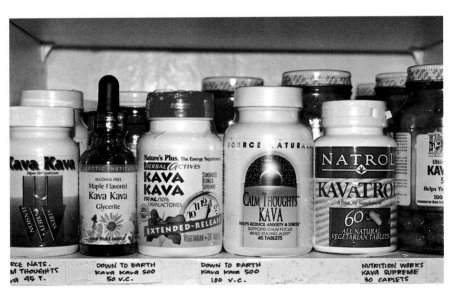

Kava is sold in natural food stores as pills, capsules, and powders. The U.S. Food and Drug Administration does not regulate kava for safety, purity, or contaminants and has not approved it as an antianxiety drug. *(Susan Scott)*

Food and Drug Administration (FDA) does not regulate kava for safety, purity, or contaminants and has not approved it as an antianxiety agent. Some Hawaiian healers warn that kava is not effective without the *mana*, or divine power, that comes with *pule*, or prayer.[4]

# Incidence

Kava is currently popular as an alternative medicine to relieve stress and anxiety. Some view it as a "natural herbal alternative to Valium, Prozac, and other mood management drugs."[5] One herbal medicine entrepreneur remarked in a 1996 *Newsweek* article, "Kava is the next big thing. We think it can be as big as coffee."[6]

In Vanuatu, Pohnpei, and other Pacific islands, kava bars proliferate and abuse is common. The potential for abuse in Hawai'i, where kava grows well, is also high.

In 1997 and 1998, the Hawaii Poison Center received no calls from people with kava exposure.

# Signs and Symptoms

Small kava doses produce a feeling of well-being and relaxation. Larger doses can cause vision disturbances, confusion, sleepiness, and decreased muscle coordination.

Researchers in Pohnpei report that drinking kava is a significant cause of severe stomach pain, particularly in people fifteen to twenty-four years old. The pain is worse when the kava is taken with alcohol. Numerous patients went to a Pohnpei emergency room complaining of severe chest pain, but no life-threatening illnesses were found. All were chronic kava drinkers, and all had consumed kava within 24 hours of experiencing the pain.[7]

Chronic drinkers of kava can have low body weight, constipation, bloodshot eyes, bad breath, shortness of breath, malnutrition, numbness, and dizziness.

Acute overdoses cause staggering gait, inability to hear, and yellow skin discoloration. Continued use produces a severe, scaly rash over the entire body. This rash resembles a cracked porcelain glaze.

Simultaneous drinking of alcohol intensifies the effects of kava.

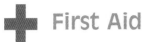

## First Aid

As with alcohol and marijuana, the symptoms of kava intoxication disappear without treatment. The time it takes to recover from kava drinking depends on the variety of kava used. Traditional users describe the potency of kava as one-day, two-day, or three-day kava. This refers to the length of time the intoxication lasts. People drinking kava should never drive a vehicle.

For acute overdoses, in which a victim cannot hear or is sedated to unconsciousness, go to an emergency room.

For stomach pain or overall illness after taking kava, stop the drug and consult a physician.

## Advanced Medical Treatment

No specific antidote or clinically useful diagnostic test exists for kava intoxication.

Kava drinking, especially with alcohol, is associated with gastritis, often presenting as severe chest pain. Scaly, yellowish skin indicates prolonged use. In one case from Germany, a woman developed acute necrotizing hepatitis after taking kava as an alternative medicine. When she stopped the kava, her liver function tests quickly became normal.[8]

The only cure for kava-induced illness is to stop drinking kava.

# LANTANA
## (Lantana camara)

*Lantana camara*, native to tropical America, has been in Hawai'i since 1858. People grow this shrub throughout the world because it flowers almost continuously and is hardy, growing well around sea spray and at high elevations. Lantana is so hardy, it has become a weed pest in the southern United States, Hawai'i, and countries including Australia, India, and South Africa. Lantana is particularly destructive because it forms thickets and inhibits the growth of other plants.

Beginning in 1902, Hawai'i officials introduced a variety of

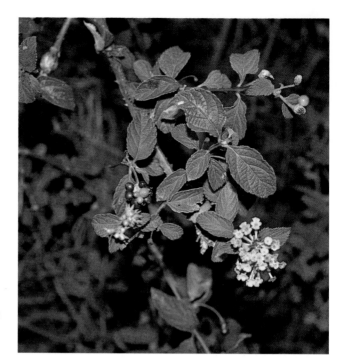

People brought lantana to Hawaiʻi as a hardy flower. It is so hardy that it proliferated throughout the Islands and has become a pesky weed. Lantana berries can be poisonous; the green ones are more toxic than the black. *(Susan Scott)*

insect species known to eat lantana seeds, flowers, stems, and leaves. Despite their efforts, lantana still grows widely throughout the Islands as a weed pest.

Lantana leaves are rough, have a strong, distinctive smell, and can cause skin rashes. The tiny berries lantana produces are delicious but poisonous when green and unripe. When ripe, the berries turn blue, then black. The toxicity of ripe berries is unknown.

## Toxin

Unripe lantana berries contain the alkaloid lantadene—a chemical that resembles atropine—and an unknown toxin. The ripe berries are far less toxic or may not be toxic at all. Some people eat ripe lantana berries as food with no ill effects. Because the reasons for this are unclear, though, it is wise to regard all berries, even black, ripe ones, as poisonous.

No human poisonings have occurred from eating lantana leaves, but cattle, sheep, buffaloes, and goats have become ill and died after eating them. An unknown substance in lantana acts as a liver toxin in livestock but not in people. The difference apparently lies in the quantity of leaves eaten and in the digestive systems of the two groups. Ruminants eat more leaves than a human would, and those leaves remain in ruminant stomachs longer than in human stomachs and thus are better absorbed.

Lantana in water can poison fish.

# Traditional and Modern Uses

In Tonga, people rub lantana leaves between their hands to produce a juice, which they drip into cuts and wounds to stop bleeding. In Malaysia and the Philippines, people use lantana as an antiseptic. In the Caribbean Islands, people make a tea from lantana leaves to cure indigestion, colds, fevers, and rheumatism.

These traditional uses of lantana are scientifically unproven and may be harmful.

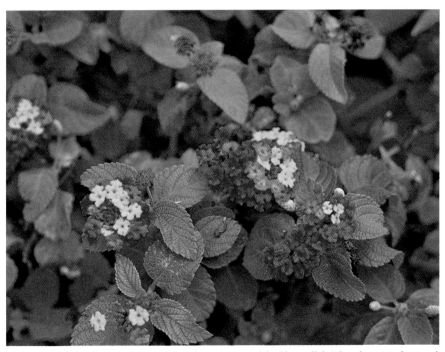

Though lantana is considered a poisonous pest in the wild, Island nurseries and plant stores still sell lantana plants in a wide variety of colors for garden use. (Susan Scott)

# Incidence

Lantana poisonings are rare in Hawai'i. In 1997 and 1998, the Hawaii Poison Center received no calls from people with lantana exposure.

In other areas, children have been poisoned from eating unripe berries; at least one died. The child was a healthy two-year-old who developed symptoms about six hours after eating unripe berries. She died about two hours later in the emergency room.

Of seventeen reported cases of people eating lantana berries, only four developed symptoms. The state of ripeness and the quantities eaten in these cases are unknown.

Since the spread of lantana throughout the world, livestock have been poisoned in nine countries over five continents.

# Signs and Symptoms

The smell of lantana can be strong enough to give some people a headache or make them feel giddy.

Lantana leaves on the skin may cause pain, itching, and redness. In the eyes, lantana can cause pain, swelling, tearing, and sensitivity to light as a result of dilated pupils.

Symptoms of eating unripe lantana berries occur from 2 1/2 to 6 hours after eating. The victim may have nausea, vomiting, diarrhea, difficulty breathing, dilated pupils, poor coordination, sleepiness, weakness, coma, and cyanosis. Death may follow.

 ## First Aid

Wash exposed skin thoroughly with soap and water. Rinse exposed eyes with tap water for at least 15 minutes. If symptoms persist after washing and rinsing, consult a doctor.

Regard the eating of any lantana berries as a serious poisoning. Even if the victim has no symptoms, go to the nearest emergency room. If symptoms have begun, or if the victim has any difficulty breathing, call 911. Take berries, flowers, and leaves of the plant to the emergency room for identification.

## Advanced Medical Treatment

No specific antidote or clinically useful diagnostic test exists for lantana berry poisoning, which presents as atropine poisoning. Make the diagnosis by physical exam and history.

A patient who has eaten lantana leaves requires no treatment other than observation.

Atropine impairs peristalsis. Therefore, if a victim has eaten any amount of ripe or unripe berries, consider emptying the stomach, even if more than an hour has elapsed since ingestion. For all ingestions, give charcoal. Catheterize for urinary retention. Use diazepam as necessary for sedation.

Consider physostigmine only for uncontrollable hyperthermia, supraventricular tachycardia with hemodynamic instability, therapy-resistant seizures, and extreme delirium. The recommended dose of physostigmine in adults is 1 to 2 milligrams intravenously over 5 minutes. Repeat every 15 minutes as needed. Never exceed 4 mg in 30 minutes.[1]

For children, start with 0.02 milligrams per kilogram, increasing dose as necessary to 0.5 mg. Repeat as needed to control symptoms. Maximum dose is 2 mg.[2]

Physostigmine dramatically reverses coma and other anticholinergic symptoms but may itself cause seizures. Never use physostigmine just to keep a patient awake.

# MANGO
## (Mangifera indica)

Mango trees, native to India, have long been grown throughout the tropics for their delicious fruit. They are so sweet, mangoes are sometimes called the king of fruits.

The trees bearing these fruits grow to about 90 feet tall, forming dense shade under thick, green leaves. Young leaves are red; crushed leaves smell like turpentine.

Don Francisco de Paula Marín, an avid horticulturist, arrived in Hawai'i from Mexico in 1791. He planted Hawai'i's first mango tree, near the corner of Vineyard and River Streets in Honolulu, sometime between 1800 and 1820. Mango trees are now common throughout the Islands in yards, gardens, and

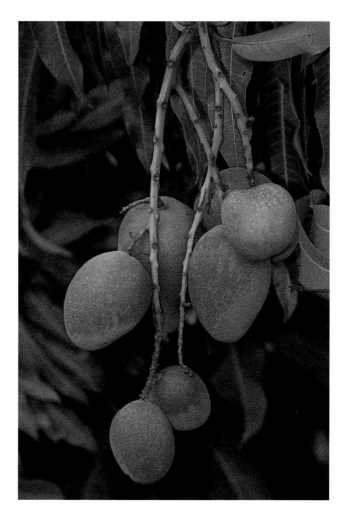

Mango trees contain a resin in the leaves, bark, and skin of the fruits. The resin is closely related to the toxin in poison ivy. Some people are allergic to this substance. *(Susan Scott)*

growing wild. They flower in January and bear fruit between March and October.

Several mango strains are good to eat and are cultivated more than others. In Hawai'i, the most common is the Hayden mango. Another popular variety is the Pirie mango.

A resin runs through the leaves, sap, and fruit skins of mango trees. Some people are allergic to this substance.

## Toxin

The leaves, sap, and fruit skin of the mango tree contain toxicodendrol, an oily resin closely related to the toxin in poison ivy. The yellow fruit inside the peelings is free of this toxin. As with poison ivy response, only some people are sensitive to this oil. Repeated exposures tend to produce worsening rashes.

The skin of unripe fruit and tree sap are the most common cause of skin rashes. When blooming, the flowers may cause breathing difficulty or swelling of the eyes and face in susceptible people.

Contrary to popular folklore, feeding various parts of mango trees to sensitive people will not give them immunity; instead, it may make them seriously ill.

## Traditional and Modern Uses

In Hawai'i, people eat mango fruit either raw or as preserves, chutney, jelly, pickles, or preserved mango seed. Woodworkers use mango wood to make bowls and other items.

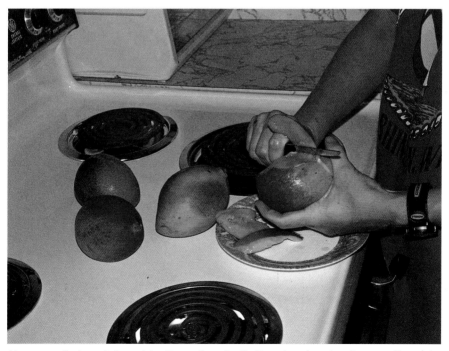

Mango resin is not found in the yellow fruit. People who develop an allergy to mango resin can still eat the fruit if someone not allergic peels it for them. Be sure and keep the peelings away from the allergic person and wash cutting boards and utensils well. *(Susan Scott)*

In Hawaiʻi, people sometimes cultivate the cashew nut tree (*Anacardium occidentale* L.), a close relative of mango. The raw juice from the shell around cashew nuts (hanging from the bottom of the fruits) causes a blistering skin rash. Cooking renders the toxin harmless but breathing fumes during the roasting process can cause an allergic reaction. Treatment for cashew rash is the same as for mango rash. The red fruits in this picture, called cashew apples, are safe to eat raw. *(Susan Scott)*

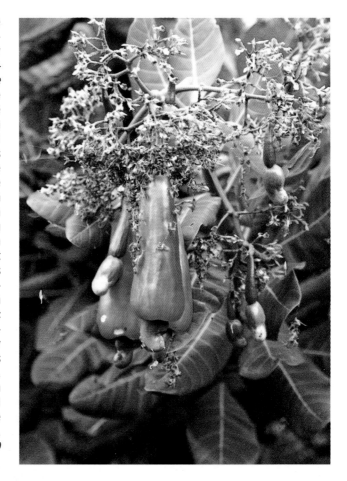

In Mexico, people use mango stems as toothbrushes. Tongans crush mango leaves with orange leaves to treat "relapse sickness," an illness they believe affects women who have just given birth or people who have recently recovered from a serious illness. In Samoa, people scrape the bark of mangoes to make a potion for coughs, sore throats, and mouth infections in babies.

Using mango as a remedy is scientifically unproven and may be harmful.

# Incidence

Most people can eat and handle mangoes with no ill effects. Some, however, can handle mangos for years, then suddenly become allergic to leaves, sap, and fruit skin. Usually, these people can still eat the yellow fruit without harm, providing someone else peels it for them.

In 1997, the Hawaii Poison Center received calls from ten people with mango rash; in 1998, six people called. These numbers likely represent only a small fraction of the mango rashes experienced by Hawai'i residents and visitors.

At least two cases, one in Hawai'i, have been reported of generalized allergic reactions after eating mangoes. At least one of these people had not handled the peel or been exposed to the sap.

# Signs and Symptoms

Rashes range from a simple, itching rash to blistering and swelling that spreads over the body. The severity of the rash depends on a person's sensitivity to the toxin.

Puffing and itching of the eyes is common. Toxin in the eyes may also cause redness, lid swelling, lid spasms, and sensitivity to light. Itching and burning lips may occur after eating unpeeled mango fruit.

## First Aid

Wash exposed skin thoroughly with soap and water. The type of toxin in mangoes quickly attaches to the cells of the skin, thus washing after 10 to 15 minutes does little to help lessen the severity of the rash. Rinse exposed eyes with tap water for 15 minutes. If the symptoms are unbearable, or become worse, consult a doctor.

Cool compresses or cool showers may ease some rash discomfort. For itching, try 1 percent hydrocortisone cream 4 times a day, and 1 or 2 25-milligram diphenhydramine (Benadryl) tablets every 6 hours. Diphenhydramine may cause drowsiness: Do not drive, swim, or surf after taking this medication. Give children diphenhydramine syrup, following the dosage directions on the package.

For swelling of the face, mouth, or throat, or any difficulty breathing, call 911. Take a branch from the tree, with leaves and fruit, to the emergency room for identification.

## Advanced Medical Treatment

Corticosteroids and oral antihistamines are the main treatments for mango rash. If the rash is severe, and topical steroids have brought no relief, give oral prednisone for several days.

Anaphylaxis from eating mangoes is rare but has occurred. The treatment is the same as for any other severe allergy.

# MUSHROOMS
## (Agaricales)

Mushrooms are not plants but are the fleshy fruiting bodies of the group of organisms called fungi (singular, fungus). Unlike most plants, fungi have no chlorophyll to covert sunlight energy to food. Instead, fungi obtain nutrients in one of three ways. The most common method is to grow on dead and decaying organic matter. These types of fungi, saprotrophs, make up about 94 percent of Hawai'i's mushroom species. The other 6 percent are parasites, taking their sustenance from living plant cells, and mycorrhizal mushrooms, which have a symbiotic relationship with the roots of trees.

Approximately 300 to 400 mushroom species grow in Hawai'i; to date, about 255 of them have been identified.

## Toxins

Some species of mushrooms produce toxins that are harmful when eaten. Contrary to popular belief, human skin does not absorb mushroom toxins during normal handling. Therefore, touching a mushroom that contains toxins is not harmful.

Usually, mushroom toxins are present only in small amounts. Several are potent enough, however, to produce characteristic symptoms even if the victim eats only a small amount of the mushroom. Cooking does not usually destroy mushroom toxins.

Mushroom toxins can be divided into seven groups. Two of these, monomethylhydrazine (MMH) and muscarine/histamine are not found in Hawai'i. The remaining five toxin

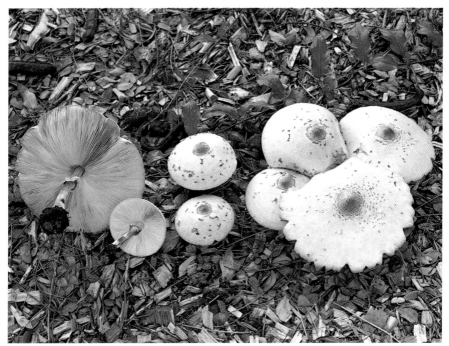

This mushroom, *Chlorophyllum molybdites*, grows on grassy lawns. The species smells and tastes good but causes vomiting and diarrhea. It is the most common source of mushroom poisoning in Hawai'i. *(Don Hemes)*

groups listed below are in descending order from the most common type of mushroom poisoning seen in Hawai'i to the least common.

### Gastrointestinal Irritants
Most of the numerous toxins in this group are still unknown. They irritate mainly the stomach and intestines, sometimes violently, but can also affect nerves and muscles. These toxins are not usually life threatening, but can be as a result of water loss.

### Hallucinogenics
The main toxins in hallucinogenic mushrooms are psilocybin, psilocin, baeocystin, norbaeocystin, and indoles similar to LSD. The effect of these toxins is mainly on the brain, causing hallucinations either pleasant or frightening. These toxins are not usually life threatening.

## Muscimol-Ibotenic Acid

Mushrooms in this category contain ibotenic acid, which the human body rapidly converts to muscimol, a chemical that inhibits nerve impulses. The effect of this and several other chemicals in these mushrooms is alternate depression and stimulation of the central nervous system. This group is also known to cause inebriation similar to alcohol inebriation.

*Amanita muscaria*, a Kaua'i species in this category, is also known to produce nausea and vomiting. Neither ibotenic acid nor muscimol, though, is known to cause these symptoms. Thus, it is likely that this mushroom contains another toxin(s) as yet unidentified.

Muscimol-ibotenic acid toxins are seldom life threatening to humans.

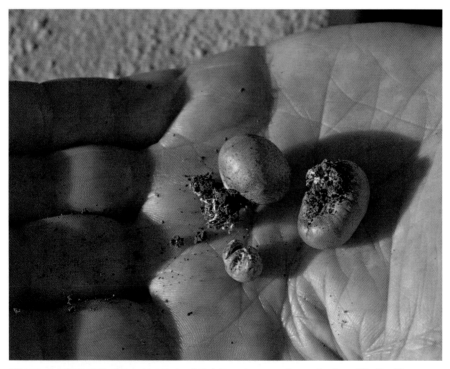

These mushrooms are a species of *Schleroderma*, also called puffballs. They are common and cause severe vomiting and diarrhea when eaten. The authors found these mushrooms at the Peacock Flats picnic ground on O'ahu's north shore. *(Susan Scott)*

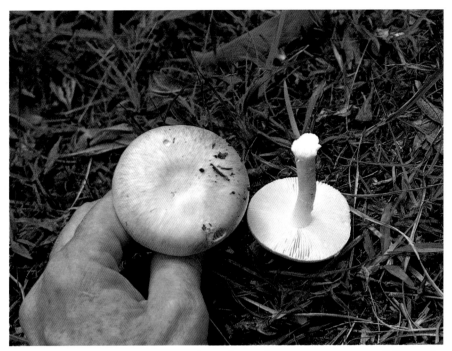

*Amanita marmorata* is an extremely toxic mushroom common on all the main Islands. Dogs have died from eating this mushroom in Hawai'i, and its toxin, a cyclopeptide, has been fatal to people on the mainland. This specimen was growing in the center of a hiking path in 'Aiea, O'ahu. *(Craig Thomas)*

### Cyclopeptides

This group of mushrooms contains amatoxins, chemicals that disrupt cell division by interfering with DNA and RNA. Organs with the highest rate of cell multiplication, such as the stomach and intestines, are damaged first, followed by the liver and kidneys. These toxins can be fatal.

### Coprine

Mushrooms in this group contain coprine, a chemical that inhibits the metabolism of alcohol in the body. Coprine causes illness similar to the alcohol-antabuse reaction when someone drinks alcohol within 24 hours of eating these mushrooms. This toxin is not usually life threatening. Coprine-bearing mushrooms do not cause illness in the absence of alcohol.

Depending on the species, mushrooms range in edibility from safe to deadly poisonous. The amount of toxins in a toxic species varies with size and environmental conditions. Different mushroom populations may produce different amounts of toxins. Also, one mushroom species may affect individuals differently; one person may become sick from eating it, but someone else may not develop symptoms.

# Traditional and Modern Uses

Some people like to pick mushrooms in the wild for food. Because some mushrooms are poisonous, this practice can be dangerous and even fatal to individuals not familiar with identifying the poisonous species.

It is common for some people to forage for mushrooms they believe to be hallucinogenic for the purpose of getting high. This, too, can be dangerous with a misidentification. Also, possessing hallucinogenic mushrooms is illegal in Hawai'i.

# Incidence

Collecting wild mushrooms to eat is more common on the mainland than in Hawai'i. In 1997, the Hawaii Poison Center received seventeen calls about mushroom exposure; in 1998, nineteen people called.

People occasionally mistake a poisonous mushroom species for an edible one. The following list details the five categories of mushroom poisoning seen in Hawai'i:

### Gastrointestinal Irritants

Most Hawai'i cases of mushroom poisoning are gastrointestinal irritants. The most common culprit is *Cholorophyllum molybdites*, a mushroom with greenish gills (the underside of the cap) that grows on lawns. This species smells and tastes good but causes vomiting and diarrhea, sometimes violent. Most people recover from eating this mushroom, but it has caused deaths in small children.

Around 1990, approximately eight female pineapple workers were treated for nausea and vomiting from mushroom poisoning. They went to an O'ahu emergency room at 2 A.M. At midnight, the workers had eaten stew containing wild mushrooms collected by one of the women. Because all the stew was gone, identifying the culprit mushroom was impossible. The women received charcoal and all recovered with no further treatment.

### Hallucinogenics

The second most common cause of mushroom poisoning in Hawai'i is from so-called magic mushrooms eaten intentionally for a mind-altering experience. The most commonly occurring species in Hawai'i is *Copelandia cyanescens*, a mushroom that grows on cow dung. Fatality from this species on the U.S. mainland is less than 1 percent.

### Muscimol-Ibotenic Acid Group

Hawai'i has at least one species from this group, *Amanita muscaria*, which has been found growing only under pines on Kaua'i. People usually eat mushrooms in this group for mind-altering experiences that are similar to alcohol inebriation.

Because muscimol and ibotenic acid are toxic to the housefly, people have used *Amanita muscaria* as an insecticide since the thirteenth century. This mushroom is therefore known as fly agaric. The species also has been used in religious ceremonies in India, Siberia, and possibly other parts of the world.

### Cyclopeptides

Hawai'i hosts at least one species from this group, *Amanita marmorata*. Two dogs on the island of Hawai'i died a day after eating this mushroom. A woman on the island of Hawai'i ate a piece of this mushroom the size of her fingernail and experienced bloody vomiting and bloody diarrhea for 48 hours. She recovered. This extremely toxic mushroom is common on all the main Islands.

The mortality rate from this species on the U.S. mainland is 20 to 30 percent. With early, appropriate intensive care, mortality may be less than 5 percent.

### Coprines

Hawai'i hosts several species of *Coprinus*, the genus that contains coprine. No cases of this type of poisoning have been recorded in Hawai'i.

# Signs and Symptoms

The toxicity of mushrooms can vary widely from species to species and from person to person. In a group of people all eating the same kind of mushroom, some may become violently ill while others have no symptoms.

Though there is some overlap, each type of mushroom toxin has its own classic symptoms.

### Gastrointestinal Irritants
• Symptoms usually begin 15 minutes to 2 hours after eating.
• Classic symptoms: nausea, vomiting, diarrhea, and abdominal cramps.
• Other symptoms: numbness and muscle spasms.
• Symptoms usually disappear in 3 to 4 hours without treatment. Full recovery is usually in 1 to 2 days. Mushrooms in this group have caused death in small children from fluid loss.

### Hallucinogenics
• Symptoms usually begin 30 to 60 minutes after eating, but occasionally begin as late as 3 hours after eating.
• Classic symptoms: Muscle relaxation, fast heartbeat, dilated pupils, dry mouth, nausea, vomiting, and hallucinations.
• Other symptoms: Mood alterations, poor coordination, dizziness, numbness, weakness, and drowsiness. Children may have fever and seizures.
• Symptoms usually disappear in 4 to 6 hours without treatment. Flashback hallucinations have occurred 2 to 3 weeks after eating the mushroom.
• "Street" mushrooms may have been laced with LSD or other drugs, making symptoms variable and confusing.

### Muscimol-Ibotenic Acid
• Symptoms begin 30 to 90 minutes after eating and peak in 2 to 3 hours.
• Classic symptoms: Intoxication resembling alcohol intoxication, periods of "highs" alternating with periods of "lows," muscle spasms and delirium followed by deep sleep from which the patient can be aroused only with difficulty. During this phase, pulse, blood pressure, and breathing are normal for deep sleep. In the mushroom *Amanita muscaria*, so far found only on Kaua'i, classic symptoms also include nausea and vomiting.
• Other symptoms: Confusion, euphoria, delusions, and dizziness. Coma is rare and seizures are rare, except in children.
• Symptoms disappear in 4 to 8 hours without treatment.

### Cyclopeptides

- One mushroom, *Amanita marmorata*, containing this deadly toxin is common throughout the main Islands, but poisonings from it are extremely rare.
- First symptoms begin 6 to 24 hours after eating.
- Classic early symptoms: Severe nausea, vomiting, headache, abdominal pain, and muscle aches.
- Later symptoms (sometimes 3 to 5 days later, after a period of well-being—the "honeymoon" phase): Abdominal pain, lack of urine production from kidney failure, yellow skin and eyes from liver failure, and seizures, followed by death.

### Coprine

- Symptoms begin 20 minutes to 2 hours after drinking alcohol within 24 hours of eating the mushroom.
- Classic symptoms: Flushing of face and neck, swelling and numbness of hands and feet, metallic taste, fast heart rate, and chest pain.
- Other symptoms: Nausea, vomiting, and sweating. Coma in severe cases.
- Symptoms disappear in 24 hours without treatment.

# First Aid

If someone becomes ill after eating wild mushrooms, it is important for health care workers to determine which mushroom species the victim ate. Save any remaining parts of any mushrooms that might have been eaten. If no mushrooms are left, find out where the mushroom was growing, and details about its size, color, and shape.

Because the possibility exists that illness from mushroom poisoning can be serious, or even fatal, take any victim with symptoms to an emergency room. If the victim has difficulty breathing, call 911. If any remains of the mushroom are available, take them to the emergency room with you.

# Advanced Medical Treatment

No easy rules exist for identifying poisonous mushrooms.

For mushroom ingestion, have the mushroom species identified as quickly as possible by a competent mycologist. The

Hawaii Poison Center has the names of specialists willing to help.

To help identify which type of mushroom the victim has eaten, ask the following questions:

- What time did the victim(s) eat the mushrooms?
- How soon did the symptoms begin?
- Did the victim drink any alcohol with 24 hours of the mushroom ingestion?
- Was more than one kind of mushroom eaten?
- Are other people who ate the mushrooms ill?
- Are other people who did not eat the mushrooms ill?
- Where was the mushroom growing?
- What was the mushroom growing on (wood, cow dung, soil, etc.)?

Give charcoal to all mushroom ingestion victims. Once the type of mushroom is determined, treat as follows:

## Gastrointestinal Irritants
Replace fluids and electrolytes as needed. Perform routine liver and kidney function tests to determine if cyclopeptide poisoning may be involved.

## Hallucinogenics
Calm patient's fears by talking calmly in a quiet room. This poisoning can usually be managed without drugs. Use diazepam as needed for agitation or seizures.

## Muscimol-Ibotenic Acid
Admit for observation all victims with symptoms. This poisoning can usually be managed without drugs. Use diazepam as needed for agitation or seizures.

## Cyclopeptides
Regard any unidentified mushroom poisoning having onset of symptoms 6 hours or more after ingestion as the highly toxic cyclopeptides. Admit the patient for monitoring and observation. Replace fluids, glucose, and electrolytes as needed. Animal experiments suggest penicillin (up to 1 million units/kilogram/day), silibilin (not generally available in the United States), or cimetidine may block the toxins' entry into

the liver. No treatment provides clinically proven benefits. Consider extracorporeal hemoperfusion over resin filters within 1 week of known ingestion.

Be prepared for hepatic or renal failure as long as 2 weeks after ingestion.

### Coprine

Replace fluids and electrolytes as needed.

This poisoning is self-limited and occurs only if the victim also drank alcohol.

# NIGHTSHADE
## (*Solanum* species)

The group of plants known as nightshade contains about 1,700 species. Hawai'i has four native species of *Solanum*, all called *pōpolo*. Three of these are relatively rare but one, *S. americanum*, is a weed common in pastures and other disturbed areas. Known as glossy or black nightshade, it bears three-eighths-inch, sweet, black berries and is the most common of the native species. Glossy nightshade is native to most Pacific islands and other tropical areas. The species most people call deadly nightshade, *Solanum dulcamara*, does not grow in Hawai'i.

The Hawaiian name for several types of introduced nightshade plants is also *pōpolo*. At least thirteen *Solanum* species have been introduced to Hawai'i. Some of these plants are familiar, nontoxic food plants, such as the potato *(S. tuberosum)*, from the Andes, and eggplant *(S. melongena)*, from Southeast Asia. Others, including the following three plants introduced as ornamentals, are not edible because they bear toxins.

• Apple of Sodom *(Solanum linnaeanum)* or *pōpolo kīkānia*. *Lei* makers sometimes use the 2-inch, yellow fruits of this African native in *lei*.

• Jerusalem cherry *(Solanum pseudocapsicum)*. This plant, probably native to Argentina, is usually grown as a potted plant for its attractive fruit.

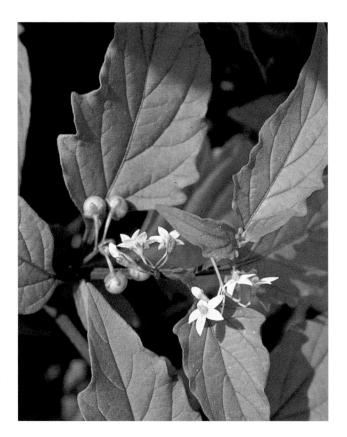

Glossy nightshade, commonly known as *pōpolo* in Hawai'i, is native to Hawai'i and other Pacific islands. The green, unripe berries are poisonous, especially to children. *(Art Whistler)*

• Cockroach berry *(Solanum capsicoides)*, or *kīkānia lei* or *akaaka*. This native of Brazil has 1-inch red fruits, also sometimes used in *lei*.

These three alien plants, along with the native species, glossy nightshade, are weeds in pastures, trails, and along roadsides throughout Hawai'i.

## Toxins

The common toxin in *Solanum* species is the glycoside solanine. Solanine damages the lining of the digestive tract and can also depress the central nervous system, thus slowing the heart rate and lowering blood pressure.

Several alkaloids are also found in some of these plants. One of them, atropine, is a chemical that affects the central nervous system.

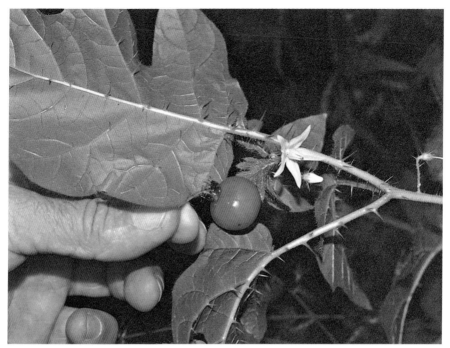

The Jerusalem cherry contains a toxin that acts directly on the heart. In Hawai'i, the Jerusalem cherry is usually grown as a potted plant. *(Susan Scott)*

The combination of these toxins can lead to confusing and contradictory symptoms, appearing one after another. For example, solanine can cause people to salivate excessively, but atropine causes dry mouth.

The Jerusalem cherry contains the alkaloid solanocapsine, a toxin that acts directly on the heart, causing slowing of the heart rate and weakening of the heart muscle.

The type and amount of toxins in the *Solanum* group vary widely from one species to another, from plant to plant, and even from part of one plant to another. For instance, the leaves, stems, and green sprouts of potatoes are poisonous but the potato itself is not.

# Traditional and Modern Uses

Ancient Hawaiians found *pōpolo (Solanum americanum)* leaves widely useful. To prevent bloating, people ate young leaves with a meal. Hawaiian healers prescribed *pōpolo* leaves, either

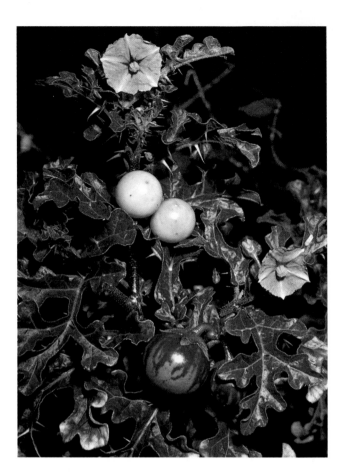

These poisonous fruits, called apple of Sodom, are about 2 inches wide. *(Art Whistler)*

cooked or raw, to treat coughs, and applied mashed leaf poultices to inflamed eyes. Pounded with salt, *pōpolo* leaves were placed on wounds to promote healing. Juice of the *pōpolo* was used as a mild laxative. It was also rubbed onto sore tendons. Either as food or tea, *pōpolo* was regarded as a good tonic, a pick-me-up.

In Tonga and the Cook Islands, people place the crushed *Solanum* leaves on mosquito bites and boils.

These traditional uses of *Solanum* plants are scientifically unproven and may be harmful.

In ancient Hawai'i, pregnant women were encouraged to eat greens, particularly *pōpolo* leaves; *pōpolo* berries were an important famine food. The blackish purple berries were also used in dyes.

# Incidence

In 1997, the Hawaii Poison Center received calls from two people exposed to nightshade species; in 1998, two people called. These numbers likely represent only a fraction of the number of nightshade exposures experienced by Hawai'i residents and visitors.

Solanine appears to have little effect on adults, but children have become ill in Florida after eating unripe glossy nightshade berries. The green berries have also caused illness and death in rabbits, cattle, sheep, goats, pigs, horses, and domestic fowl. In Hawai'i, people often eat the ripe, tasty black berries of this plant with no ill effects. The leaves and unripe berries, though, may be mildly poisonous.

Though rare, deaths have been reported in Brazil and New Zealand from children eating unripe (green) Jerusalem cherries.

# Signs and Symptoms

Symptoms from eating *Solanum* plants range from none to severe in the digestive and/or nervous systems.

Sometimes, symptoms begin within one-half hour of eating the plant. Other times, symptoms of poisoning do not appear for up to 24 hours.

Digestive symptoms include excessive salivation, a scratchy throat, stomach irritation or cramps, vomiting, and diarrhea. Diarrhea can last 3 to 6 days.

Symptoms of nervous system involvement vary widely and can include dilated pupils and a giddy, delirious, or drowsy victim. Further nervous system symptoms can include trembling, unsteady gait, weakness, headache, loss of speech or consciousness, and dry mouth, throat, and skin. Acute poisoning can cause seizures and respiratory paralysis. Symptoms may persist for days.

 ## First Aid

Adults with nausea, vomiting, or diarrhea after eating any *Solanum* plant should drink lots of fluids to replace water lost. If diarrhea persists, or nervous system symptoms appear, go to an emergency room.

Because children are more susceptible to solanine poisoning than adults, those suspected of eating any part of these plants should be taken to an emergency room.

If either an adult or child has difficulty breathing, or collapses, call 911. Take flowers, stems, fruits, and leaves of the plant to the emergency room for identification.

## Advanced Medical Treatment

No specific antidote or clinically useful diagnostic test exists for solanine poisoning, which is easily mistaken for viral or bacterial gastroenteritis. Make the diagnosis by physical exam and history. Use antiemetics as needed. Replace fluids and electrolytes. Atropine may be needed for symptomatic bradycardia.

Poisoning from this group of plants may also present as atropine poisoning. Atropine impairs peristalsis. Therefore, in severe poisonings consider emptying the stomach even if more than an hour has elapsed since ingestion. For all ingestions, give charcoal. Catheterize for urinary retention. Use diazepam as necessary for sedation.

Consider physostigmine only for uncontrollable hyperthermia, supraventricular tachycardia with hemodynamic instability, therapy-resistant seizures, and extreme delirium. The recommended dose of physostigmine in adults is 1 to 2 milligrams intravenously over 5 minutes. Repeat every 15 minutes as needed. Never exceed 4 mg in 30 minutes.[1]

For children, start with 0.02 milligrams per kilogram, increasing dose as necessary to 0.5 mg. Repeat as needed to control symptoms. Maximum dose is 2 mg.[2]

Physostigmine dramatically reverses coma and other anticholinergic symptoms, but may mask solanine symptoms in mixed poisonings. Physostigmine may also cause seizures. Never use physostigmine just to keep a patient awake.

# OLEANDER
## (Nerium oleander)

Oleander shrubs are native to the Mediterranean and other warm areas from Iran to Japan. They are popular ornamental

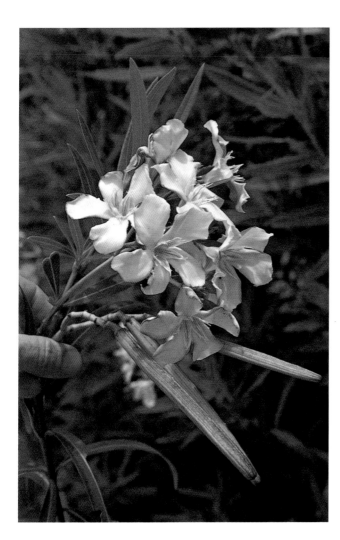

Oleander bushes grow in yards, parks, and along highways throughout Hawai'i. The shrubs are deadly poisonous, a fact apparently known to most people, since oleander poisonings in Hawai'i are rare. *(Susan Scott)*

trees in Hawai'i, Florida, and the tropics because their lovely pink, white, and red flowers break down quickly when they fall and do not need to be raked up. Also, oleanders are resistant to insect pests and grow well in sunny regions, requiring no more water than the grass they grow in.

The one major drawback of cultivating oleander shrubs and trees is that the entire plant is deadly poisonous, containing a heart toxin that can easily kill people.

Despite this, oleanders are extremely common in Hawai'i, growing on median strips, in parks, and as borders along yards.

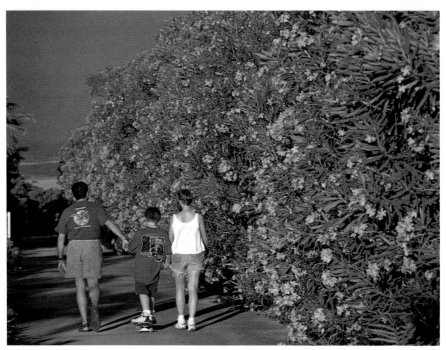

Pink oleander is one of the most common varieties. All parts of the oleander bush—seed pods, leaves, flowers, and branches—are toxic. Never cook food over an oleander wood fire or skewered on oleander sticks. *(Susan Scott)*

# Toxin

All parts of the oleander plant contain neriin and oleandrin, two potent cardiac glycosides. Cardiac glycosides block normal electrical impulses throughout the body, including the heart, by interfering with the exchange of sodium and potassium in and out of nerve and muscle cells.

Oleander also contains a substance that can irritate the mucus membrane of the mouth, but it does not often cause skin rashes.

Inhaling oleander plant dust while raking the leaves may irritate the nose and throat. Inhaling smoke from burning oleander trees can cause poisoning, as does eating food cooked on an oleander stick. Drinking vase water from cut oleander flowers can cause death.

People experience a wide range of responses after eating plants containing cardiac glycosides. Some barely become sick;

others have died. Regard all parts of this plant—whether green, dry, or burning—as extremely toxic. Never use an oleander stick to roast marshmallows or hot dogs.

## Traditional and Modern Uses

Extracts of oleander are used in Turkey as a cancer treatment. It is not the cardiac glycosides that act against the cancer but rather a carbohydrate found in the plant. Research is ongoing as to the effectiveness of this treatment.

In North Africa, some people attribute magical powers to an oleander plant when the leaves grow in four pairs around the stalk.

In India, people once used oleander extract to treat Hansen's disease (leprosy). They also used it to induce abortions and as a paste to kill lice and other vermin. Such traditional uses of this plant are scientifically unproven and extremely dangerous. Some may cause death.

In Sanskrit, the name for the oleander plant means horse killer.

## Incidence

Though the oleander tree is common in Hawai'i, poisonings from it are rare. Apparently, most people in the state are aware of the plant's toxicity. In 1997, the Hawaii Poison Center received calls from two people exposed to oleander; in 1998, six people called.

Not everyone, however, knows about the dangers of oleander. A thirty-year-old woman in California died about ten hours after drinking tea made from oleander leaves she thought were eucalyptus leaves. In India, children have died from eating oleander flowers.

In Florida, children have developed symptoms of heart failure after merely licking the tree's sap from their fingers.

People have become ill with oleander poisoning from arranging a bouquet of oleander flowers; juice from the flowers got on a woman's fingers and later, when she smoked a cigarette, came in contact with her lips. A Miami woman attempted suicide by soaking twelve oleander leaves in water overnight, then drinking the water. She nearly died.

People in Hawai'i have become ill from eating food cooked

with oleander branches in Hawaiian ovens. One person died after eating meat that was skewered on an oleander branch and cooked over an open fire.

## Signs and Symptoms

People who eat any part of an oleander plant may experience immediate burning, redness, and swelling of the lips and mouth.

Swallowing this plant can cause the victim to have nausea, vomiting, abdominal pain, and cramping. This can go on for several hours before the generalized heart symptoms begin, which include slow or irregular heartbeat, dizziness, headache, and confusion. Victims may feel drowsy or giddy.

## First Aid

Regard as a medical emergency the swallowing of any part of this plant, inhaling smoke from it, or eating food cooked on its branches. Call 911. Take flowers, leaves, and a branch from the tree to the emergency room for identification.

## Advanced Medical Treatment

The effects of the cardiac glycocides neriin and oleandrin are similar to digoxin and digitoxin. Therefore, laboratory tests for these drugs may be positive for some (but not all) oleander poisonings. Because these tests rely on cross-reactivity between the plant's cardiac glycosides and digoxin or digitoxin, serum levels do not necessarily correlate with biological activity. A low digoxin or digitoxin level may indicate a potentially fatal level of oleander cardiac glycosides.

An elevated potassium level in the presence of a plant inges-tion suggests cardiac glycoside exposure.

If the patient has swallowed oleander an hour or less before going to the ER, empty the stomach. For all patients suspected of eating oleander, regardless of time elapsed, give charcoal.

Victims suspected of eating plants containing cardiac glyco-sides require cardiac monitoring. However, the effect of cardiac glycosides on the heart may be delayed; monitor asymptomatic patients for at least 12 hours before discharge.

For life-threatening arrythmias, hyperkalemia, prolonged PR

intervals, widened QRS segments, or altered mental status, administer 10 vials of digoxin immune FAB intravenously. In one case of cardiac glycoside poisoning from oleander, the patient woke up 4 minutes after FAB treatment was started, and his potassium level normalized in 1 hour. If improvement is minimal, give another 10 vials. The cross-reactivity for binding may require a high concentration of digoxin immune FAB.

The risks of digoxin immune FAB include fever, apnea, hypokalemia, and hypoglycemia. Rebound toxicity occurs in 3 to 11 days in a small fraction of patients treated with digoxin immune FAB. Some researchers suggest a continuous FAB infusion after an initial bolus. Hemoperfusion and forced diuresis are of no benefit.

If FAB is not available, use IV atropine to treat bradycardia, and use lidocaine, amiodarone, or phenytoin for ventricular arrythmias. Consider phenytoin or a pacemaker in victims with second- or third-degree heart block.

# PENCIL PLANT, CROWN OF THORNS, RED SPURGE, AND SLIPPER FLOWER
## (*Euphorbia* and *Pedilanthus* species)

The pencil plant *(Euphorbia tirucalli)* is a native of Africa. Pencil plants are interesting because their rubbery, green branches have no leaves, or only a few tiny ones, making them look like fantastic stick trees.

A close relative of the pencil plant is the crown of thorns *(Euphorbia milli)*, a native of Madagascar. This prickly ornamental produces lovely flowers year-round; most are red but some are pink, orange, yellow, or cream colored. Legend has it that these flowers were white until they were used to fashion the crown placed on Christ's head before his crucifixion. After that, the flowers turned and remained red.

Red spurge *(Euphorbia cotinifolia)* is a native tree of Central and South America that grows to about 25 feet tall. It has maroon or ruby red leaves, red branchlets, and tiny white flowers.

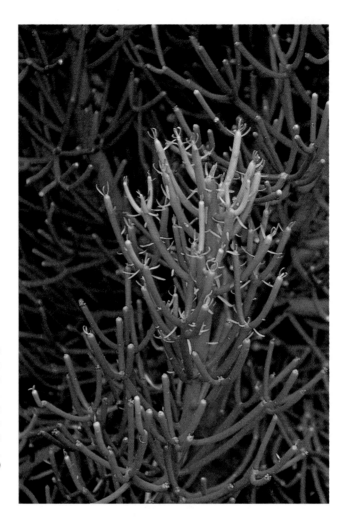

Pencil plants are harmless when intact. When broken, however, the stems ooze a thick, white sap that can irritate the skin and eyes. *(Craig Thomas)*

The slipper flower *(Pedilanthus tithymaloides)* is a succulent ornamental plant that gets it name from half-inch-long, shoe-shaped flowers. This plant is native to northern South America and the Caribbean Islands.

All four of these species are popular in Hawai'i as garden and houseplants despite their milky, rash-inducing juice.

## Toxin

The juice from these species contains euphorbol and other terpenes, chemicals that can irritate the eyes, skin, and stomach, mildly to severely depending on the species, the

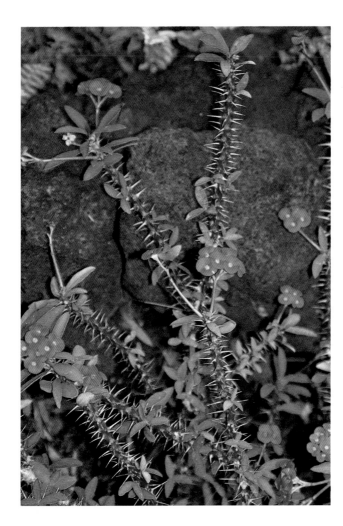

Crown of thorns plants can be formidable to tend. Besides the danger of being pricked by their sharp thorns, the stems, when broken or scratched, ooze a white sap that can cause a rash. *(Craig Thomas)*

amount of sap involved, and the length of contact. The thick, white sap from these plants oozes quickly from breaks or even scratches in the stems.

## Traditional and Modern Uses

People in Africa grow pencil plants as hedges to keep animals in or people out. Healers in Asia and Africa use pencil plant juice to treat asthma, toothaches, and general aches and pains.

Occasionally, traditional healers have used *Euphorbia* species for removal of warts, to induce vomiting, and as laxatives. The action of these plants is usually extreme.

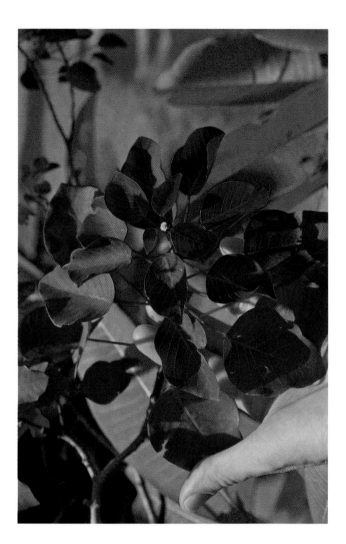

Red spurge is a hardy tree grown for its ruby-colored leaves. Sap from this plant can cause a severe rash. *(Susan Scott)*

In tropical America, people have used red spurge to stop bleeding and as arrow poison. This plant has also been used as fish poison, but it may make the fish too toxic for safe eating.

Healers in tropical America use the milky juice of slipper flower stems as a drastic remedy for some diseases.

Using any of these plants as remedies is scientifically unproven and may be harmful.

Researchers currently are using several *Euphorbia* plants in the study of skin cancers. Some *Euphorbia* plants are effective against leukemia.

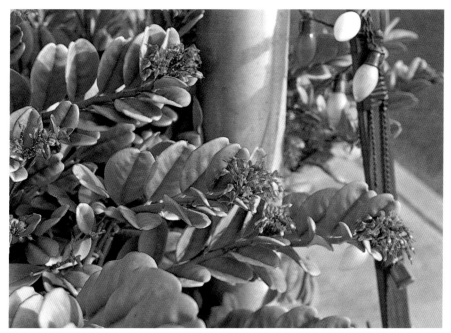

Slipper flower stems contain a white sap that is often irritating to skin and eyes. These are popular garden plants because of their dainty, slipperlike flowers. *(Susan Scott)*

# Incidence

These plants are common in Hawai'i's yards and gardens. Accidental skin and eye exposures thus are fairly common, especially during trimming and pruning sessions. When cut or broken, these plant stems quickly ooze white sap. Children have been known to drink dripping juice from pencil plants, thinking they are drinking milk from a tree.

In 1997 and 1998, the Hawaii Poison Center received no calls from people with crown of thorns, red spurge, or slipper flower exposures. In 1997, the center received calls from six people exposed to pencil plant sap; in 1998, seven people called.

These numbers likely represent only a small fraction of pencil plant and other *Euphorbia* exposures experienced by Hawai'i residents and visitors. Gardeners are sometimes exposed on the face and in the eyes by wiping them with contaminated fingers or gloves. Occasionally, when someone snaps off a branch from one of these plants, either accidentally or purposely, they are sprayed with sap.

# Signs and Symptoms

Juice in the eye can cause intense pain, redness and tearing, ulcers on the surface of the eye, and temporary blindness. Irritation of the eyes may take a month or more to disappear.

On the skin, juice from these plants can cause redness and swelling 2 to 8 hours after exposure. Blisters may form, reaching their peak in 4 to 12 hours. The severity of the rash depends on how much of the milky juice was on the skin and how long it stayed there. Skin reactions usually fade in 3 to 4 days, leaving no marks.

Inhaling the dust of these dried plants can irritate the nose and lungs, causing sneezing and/or coughing.

Eating any part of these four plants may cause a burning sensation on the lips, mouth, tongue, and throat. Swallowing the plant can cause severe stomach pain, vomiting, and diarrhea. Severe internal poisoning is extremely rare.

 ## First Aid

Rinse eyes exposed to juice from these plants immediately with tap water for 15 minutes. Wash exposed skin as quickly as possible with soap and water. Speed is important because the longer the contact, the worse the symptoms.

For itching, try 1 percent hydrocortisone cream 4 times a day, and 1 or 2 25-milligram diphenhydramine (Benadryl) tablets every 6 hours. Diphenhydramine may cause drowsiness: Do not drive, swim, or surf after taking this medication. Give children diphenhydramine syrup, following the dosage directions on the package.

For hives, persistent rash, or unbearable eye irritation, go to an emergency room. For facial swelling, any difficulty breathing, or collapse, call 911. Take stems, leaves, and flowers of the plant to the emergency room for identification.

 ## Advanced Medical Treatment

No specific antidote or diagnostic test exists for pencil plant, crown of thorns, red spurge, or slipper flower exposure. Direct treatment at relieving pain and swelling. Systemic steroids and antihistamines do not significantly relieve the discomfort from exposure to these plants.

Eye exposure can cause conjunctivitis or corneal ulceration, which responds to nonspecific treatment. There are no reports of long-term damage.

For large ingestions, give charcoal; replace fluids and electrolytes as needed.

# PERIWINKLE
## *(Catharanthus roseus)*

Periwinkles are native to Madagascar. These 1 to 2 foot–high shrubs bloom year-round and are popular as ground cover in gardens throughout tropical and subtropical areas of the world.

Periwinkles were brought to Hawai'i in the 1800s as garden plants. They escaped and have been growing wild in the Islands at least since 1871.

Periwinkle toxins rarely poison people but sometimes poison livestock. Some people call periwinkles vinca after their former scientific name, *Vinca rosea.*

## Toxin

All parts of the periwinkle contain vinblastine and vincristine, two powerful nerve toxins that cause bone marrow suppression and interfere with cell division.

These chemicals can cause deformities in the unborn children of pregnant women who eat or smoke this plant. Eating small amounts of a periwinkle plant probably is not dangerous except possibly for pregnant women.

## Traditional and Modern Uses

Vinblastine and vincristine are used in modern medicine to treat cancer. Usually, the drugs are given intravenously, as vinblastine and vincristine are absorbed poorly in the human digestive tract.

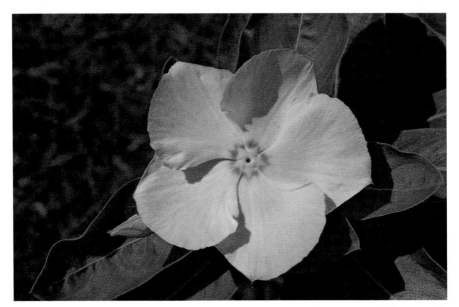

Periwinkles, commonly called vinca, are common ground-cover plants in Hawai'i. Their centers look hollow. Human poisonings from vinca are rare. More commonly, livestock suffer the consequences of the plant's two powerful nerve toxins. *(Susan Scott)*

Occasionally, people smoke periwinkle supposedly to get high. This is extremely dangerous and may result in permanent injury or even death.

## Incidence

Human poisonings from eating these plants are rare. In 1997, the Hawaii Poison Center received one call from a person with periwinkle exposure; in 1998, there were no periwinkle exposure calls. Livestock poisonings are more common.

Poisonings have occurred after people have smoked the dried leaves of this plant, presumably to get high.

## Signs and Symptoms

People do not usually eat enough of this plant to become ill.

Smoking the leaves can cause the same symptoms as an intravenous overdose of vinblastine and/or vincristine: Fever,

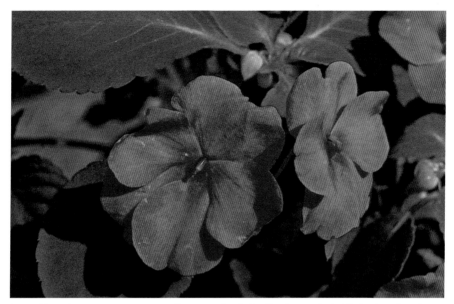

Impatiens is a common ground-cover plant similar to periwinkle but not poisonous. To tell the difference, examine the leaves and the flower centers and petals to detect the variations between the two. *(Susan Scott)*

nausea, vomiting, and stomach pain occur within the first 24 hours. Later, victims feel overall numbness and weakness followed by delirium, hallucinations, coma, and seizures. Death can occur within a week.

 ## First Aid

Wash exposed skin with soap and water. Rinse eyes exposed to periwinkle with copious amounts of tap water for at least 15 minutes. For persistent irritation, swelling, vision impairment, or pain, consult a doctor.

If someone has smoked dried periwinkle, regard it as a medical emergency. Call 911. Take the leaves and flowers to the emergency room for identification.

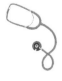 ## Advanced Medical Treatment

Irrigate eyes and wounds with copious amounts of water to prevent local and systemic symptoms.

Smoking or eating large amounts of periwinkle can produce the same symptoms as an overdose of vinblastine and vincristine. No specific antidote or diagnostic test exists for these drugs.

The initial phase requires symptomatic treatment of gastro-intestinal symptoms. Give charcoal. After the first 24 hours, life-threatening neuropathy may occur. Both vincristine and vinblastine cause bone marrow suppression.

# PLUMERIA
## (*Plumeria* species)

Plumeria trees are natives of tropical America and the West Indies, where they are often called frangipani. These trees grow easily from cuttings and are common throughout Hawai'i

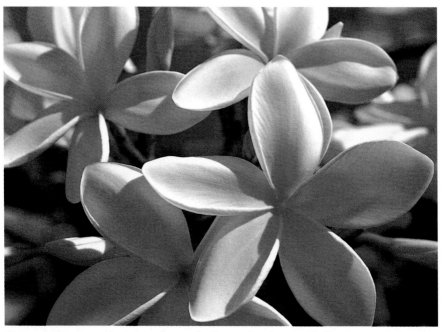

Plumeria trees are common in yards throughout Hawai'i; the fragrant flowers are common in *lei*. Plumerias rarely cause rashes or poisonings in Hawai'i. *(Susan Scott)*

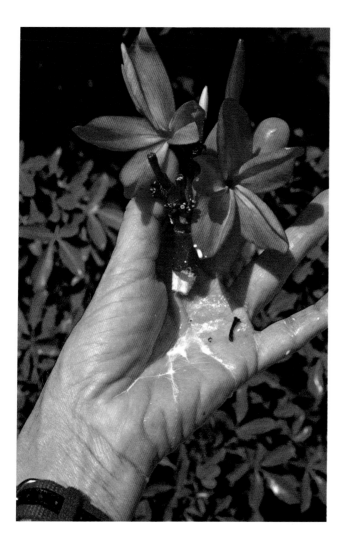

When cut, plumeria trees ooze a milky sap, harmless to most people. After taking this photo, however, the photographer developed a mild rash on several fingers. It disappeared the next day without treatment. *(Susan Scott)*

in parks, gardens, and yards. People cultivate plumeria for their fragrant yellow, white, red, and pink flowers, commonly used in *lei*.

Though some plumeria species retain their leaves year-round, most drop them in winter and grow new ones in spring. The flowers grow nearly year-round, blossoming during the winter at the branch tips of otherwise bare trees. The Hawaiian name for plumeria flowers is *pua melia*.

Most plumeria trees in Hawai'i do not produce fruit. The branches, when cut, ooze a thick, milky sap.

# Toxin

All parts of the plumeria tree contain crotinic acid, lupeol, calcium salts of plumieric acid, the cathartic plumerid, and saponins.

When eaten, these chemicals irritate the stomach and intestines. On the skin of sensitive people, they can cause a rash.

Plumeria toxins do not cause a rash in most people, and poisonings are usually mild.

# Traditional and Modern Uses

Indigenous people of South America have used plumeria as medicine to treat worm infestations and malaria. In Brazil, plumeria is used to induce menstrual flow and as a laxative.

Using plumeria as a remedy is scientifically unproven and may be harmful.

# Incidence

In 1997, the Hawaii Poison Center received calls from twenty people about contact with plumeria; in 1998, thirty-one people called. Because plumeria flowers are so common in Hawai'i, these numbers likely represent only a small fraction of plumeria exposures experienced by Hawai'i residents and visitors.

Incidents of children putting these flowers into their mouths are common. Usually, symptoms are nonexistent or mild.

People in Hawai'i have become ill after eating plumeria flowers in salads.

# Signs and Symptoms

Most people can touch plumeria flowers, branches, and sap with no symptoms. In sensitive individuals, a rash with blisters may appear on exposed skin.

People eating plumeria flowers may have vomiting and/or diarrhea several hours later. Usually, the diarrhea lasts only a few hours.

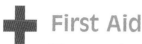 ## First Aid

Vomiting, diarrhea, and rash from contact with plumeria usually disappear without treatment.

If plumeria sap gets in the eyes, rinse with large amounts of tap water. Consult a physician if blurred vision or persistent burning develop.

For rash, wash the area thoroughly with soap and water. If itching persists, try 1 percent hydrocortisone cream 4 times a day, and 1 or 2 25-milligram diphenhydramine (Benadryl) tablets every 6 hours. Diphenhydramine may cause drowsiness: Do not drive, swim, or surf after taking this medication. Give itching children diphenhydramine syrup, following the dosage directions on the package.

For hives or persistent diarrhea, go to an emergency room. For facial swelling, any difficulty breathing, or collapse, call 911. Take flowers, stems, and leaves of the plant to the emergency room for identification.

 ## Advanced Medical Treatment

No specific antidote or clinically useful diagnostic test exists for plumeria rash or poisoning. Most cases are mild and respond to first aid.

Decontaminate skin and/or eyes. There are no reports of serious corneal injury.

Give charcoal for ingestions; replace fluids and electrolytes as needed.

# POINSETTIA
## (Euphorbia pulcherrima)

About 1,200 *Euphorbia* species grow throughout the warm regions of the world. These plants are extremely variable in form and also in toxicity. In this book, poinsettia *(Euphorbia pulcherrima)* has a separate heading from its *Euphorbia* relatives not because it is particularly lethal but because, contrary to popular belief, it is not.

Joel Poinsett, American ambassador to Mexico in 1828,

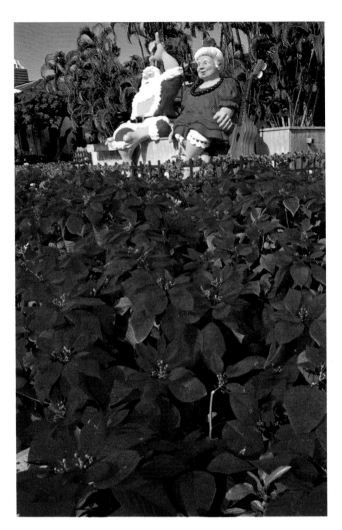

Poinsettias by the thousand adorn Honolulu Hale each Christmas season. This plant's erroneous reputation as highly poisonous resulted from a report by a Honolulu physician in 1944 stating that in 1919 a Fort Shafter two-year-old had died after eating a single poinsettia leaf. The report was never confirmed. *(Susan Scott)*

introduced poinsettias from their native Mexico to the United States. Because their floral leaves turn bright red during the flowering period, November through March, poinsettias soon became popular Christmas plants.

The lovely plant gained an undeserved bad reputation after Honolulu physician Harry Arnold wrote in 1944 that more than twenty years earlier, a Fort Shafter two-year-old had died after eating a single poinsettia leaf. Dr. Arnold later admitted he had not confirmed the supposed poinsettia-related fatality; the 1919 incident had been hearsay.

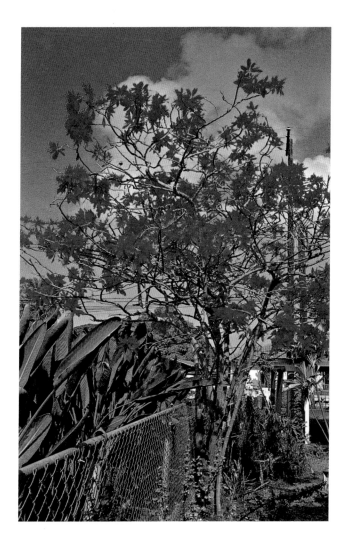

Poinsettias are popular yard trees in Hawai'i because their leaves turn red in December. Touching the plants does not usually cause a rash. Eating poinsettia leaves may cause vomiting but is not a serious poisoning. *(Susan Scott)*

The misinformation, however, lived on. At one time, citizen action groups demanded that potted poinsettia plants carry a warning label. In 1970, the FDA stated in a press release that "one poinsettia leaf can kill a child." In 1980, a North Carolina county banned the plants from nursing homes.

To this day, the myth persists that this plant is potentially deadly. It is not.

In Hawai'i, poinsettias grow to about 10 feet tall as shrubs in yards and gardens. Another species of poinsettia, *Euphorbia cyathophora*, grows wild in dry, disturbed areas.

# Toxin

Poinsettias do not contain the irritant diterpene found in many other *Euphorbia* species. Contact with poinsettias rarely causes a rash; when it does, it is usually mild. Poinsettia is not particularly irritating to the eyes. Drops of plant juice in rat eyes produced no damage.

Eating poinsettia leaves may result in vomiting but does not cause serious poisoning.

# Traditional and Modern Uses

Nursing mothers in Mexico make a tea of poinsettia leaves, believing the mixture will increase their milk flow. Healers there also apply poultices of the leaves to skin lesions.

Some American Indians reportedly used poinsettia juice to remove unwanted hair from the body. The Aztecs ate poinsettia leaves to induce abortion.

Using poinsettia as a remedy is scientifically unproven and may be harmful. Fishermen in South China use poinsettias to poison fish.

# Incidence

In 1997, the Hawaii Poison Center received calls from ten people exposed to poinsettias; in 1998, four people called. These numbers undoubtedly represent only a small number of poinsettia exposures experienced by Hawai'i residents.

From 1985 to 1992, poinsettia exposures accounted for 22,793 calls to American Poison Control Centers. There were no fatalities. Of these calls, 96 percent of the callers were not seen by a doctor and 92 percent had no symptoms from the plant.

Most cases of leaves eaten involved children under five, from December through February. The bright red holiday plants are often within reach of children and tempting to touch.

Of the 1,129 cases of skin exposure, only six people had moderate rashes; none had a severe rash.

Gardeners who work with poinsettias sometimes develop allergic skin rashes after frequent contact with the plant.

# Signs and Symptoms

Poinsettia juice in the eyes has little effect beyond minor pain, redness, and tearing.

On the skin, poinsettia leaves and juice may cause mild redness. In particularly sensitive people, swelling and blisters may develop.

Eating poinsettia may cause irritation of the mouth. An eight-month-old found chewing on a leaf had burns at the corners of the mouth. Five to 20 percent of poinsettia ingestions cause nausea, vomiting, or diarrhea. This usually stops soon on its own.

 ## First Aid

Rinse eyes exposed to poinsettia juice with tap water for 15 minutes. Wash exposed skin thoroughly with soap and water. If irritation or pain persists, consult a doctor.

Mouth and skin blisters and/or vomiting after eating poinsettia leaves disappear without treatment. For severe blisters, hives, or persistent vomiting and diarrhea, go to an emergency room. For facial swelling, any difficulty breathing, or collapse, call 911. Take leaves and flowers of the plant to the emergency room for identification.

 ## Advanced Medical Treatment

No specific antidote or diagnostic test exists for poinsettia exposure. Most cases cause little if any reaction and require no treatment. Vomiting is usually self-limited and not extensive enough to warrant fluid and electrolyte replacement.

# POKEBERRY AND CORAL BERRY
## (*Phytolacca* species and *Rivina humilis*)

Hawai'i hosts three species of pokeberry. One, *pōpolo kū mai* (*Phytolacca sandwicensis*), is native to the Islands, growing wild in damp forests and along streambeds. It reaches about 4 feet tall as a shrub or trailing bush. A similar species is the southern

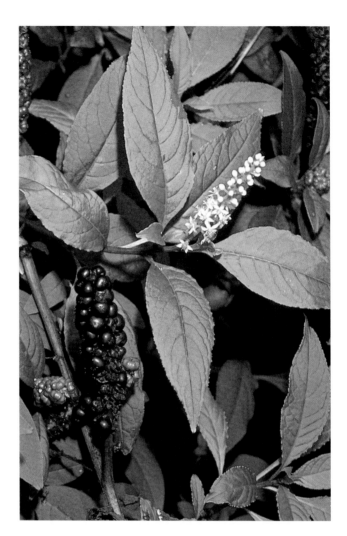

Ancient Hawaiians used dark purple pokeberries as tattoo dye. The berries are better suited to use as dye than as food because they sometimes make people seriously ill. *(Art Whistler)*

pokeberry *(Phytolacca octandra)*, native to tropical America. It, too, grows wild throughout the Islands and can thrive in either wet or dry areas. Hawai'i's third pokeberry, the ombu tree *(Phytolacca dioica)*, is a fast-growing tree from South America grown in parks and yards for shade. It grows to 50 feet tall and can have a trunk diameter of 3 feet. Pokeberries of all these species are dark purple, about the size of blueberries.

A close relative of the pokeberry plant is the coral berry or rouge plant *(Rivina humilis)*. This 3-foot-tall plant, native from Florida to South America, now grows wild in Hawai'i in

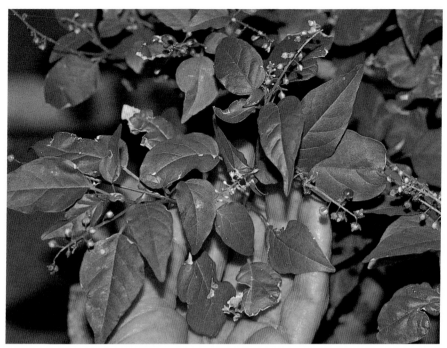

Like pokeberries, coral berries can be dangerous eating. The tiny coral berries, the size of a peppercorn or smaller, can be red, like these, or orange. *(Susan Scott)*

shaded, disturbed areas. Coral berries are either red or orange and are about the size of peppercorns, or smaller.

The root, leaves, berries, and seeds of all these plants bear various amounts of toxins.

# Toxin

Pokeberry and coral berry roots, leaves, berries, and seeds contain the toxic alkaloid phytolaccine and other triterpene toxins. These toxins irritate the digestive system and can affect the central nervous system. Triterpene toxins also impair red blood cell formation and damage mature red blood cells.

The highest concentration of toxins is in the roots, followed by the leaves, then the stems, then the unripe berries.

Boiling twice (and discarding the water each time) supposedly destroys the toxins and makes the leaves, shoots, and

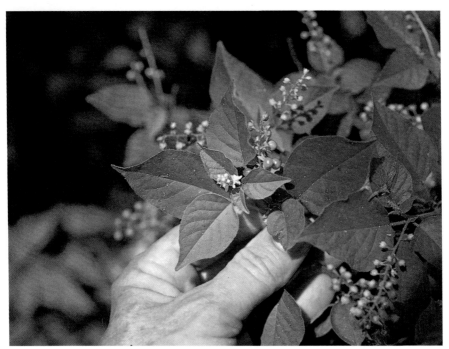

These orange coral berries are the same species *(Rivina humilis)* as the red ones. *(Susan Scott)*

roots safe to eat, but people have experienced symptoms even after this careful preparation. Though ripe berries are the least toxic part of the plant, people have become ill after eating them.

The toxins can enter the body directly and cause symptoms if berry juice gets into open wounds.

## Traditional and Modern Uses

Ancient Hawaiians used native pokeberry juice for tattoo dye. After embedding shark teeth or sharp shells in a flat board, they dipped the teeth or shells in a pokeberry mixture and struck the person with the board. The wounds healed with a permanent stain.

The English have grown coral berries in greenhouses for two centuries as dye plants. In other parts of the world, cooks use the berries in pies.

In the southern United States, people eat the young shoots

of pokeberry plants as greens (after thorough cooking). This popular, traditional dish is called poke salad.

People in several countries use pokeberry as medicine. American Indians made a salve of powdered pokeberry root for skin ailments. Traditional healers still use the roots and berries as medicine for skin diseases, eye irritation, aches and pains, and indigestion. These medicines can be in the form of tea.

In Mexico, people use coral berries as a dye and as medicine, and the leaves to treat colds and heal wounds.

Using coral berries or pokeberries as a remedy is scientifically unproven and may be harmful.

# Incidence

Pokeberry and coral berry poisoning in Hawai'i is rare. In 1997 and 1998, the Hawaii Poison Center received no calls from people with pokeberry or coral berry exposure.

People have died from eating pokeberry greens, either undercooked or when a portion of the roots were accidentally included in the pot. Others have become ill even when the greens were properly prepared. A two-year-old died from eating pokeberries. In a separate incident, a five-year-old died after drinking pokeberries that had been crushed and added to sugar and water to simulate grape juice.

People have become ill after eating pigeons that fed on pokeberries. Fatalities have occurred from overdoses prescribed by traditional healers.

People usually become poisoned after eating uncooked pokeberry leaves in salads or mistaking the root for an edible vegetable.

# Signs and Symptoms

People with pokeberry poisoning have a burning sensation in the mouth and stomach, then violent vomiting and severe diarrhea, often foamy and sometimes bloody. These symptoms occur from 1/2 hour to 5 1/2 hours after eating and can last up to two days.

The toxins can also cause headache, sweating, excessive salivation, sore throat, blurred vision, and, rarely, temporary blindness. In severe poisonings, victims may have weakness, excessive yawning, slowed breathing, fast heartbeat, dizziness, seizures, and coma, and may die.

## First Aid

Pokeberry juice can be absorbed in a cut or through abraded skin. Wash the exposed area thoroughly with soap and water. Go to an emergency room if pain persists in the cut or if symptoms of poisoning appear.

Pokeberry and coral berry poisoning can be life threatening. Take a victim showing symptoms to an emergency room. For facial swelling, any difficulty breathing, or collapse, call 911. Take berries, leaves, seeds, roots, and/or stems of the plant to the emergency room for identification.

## Advanced Medical Treatment

No specific antidote or diagnostic test exists for pokeberry or coral berry poisoning. Look for purple or reddish stains on the hands, face, and tongue for diagnosis.

Direct treatment at controlling emesis. Give charcoal; replace fluids and electrolytes if needed. Rarely, patients have an altered level of consciousness; be prepared to protect the airway. No treatment prevents hemolysis.

# STAR-OF-BETHLEHEM
## (Hippobroma longiflora)

Star-of-Bethlehem was originally native to the Caribbean Islands but is now a weed throughout the tropics, including Hawai'i. It has been in the Islands at least since 1864; it grows wild in disturbed areas with moderate rainfall.

This weed grows 1 to 2 feet tall and bears white, star-shaped flowers. The Hawaiian name, *pua hōkū*, means star flower.

The leaf edges of this plant bear menacing-looking toothed points. Though the star-of-Bethlehem has no visible thorns, beware of even touching the leaves, stems, or flowers. The sap is extremely irritating and toxic.

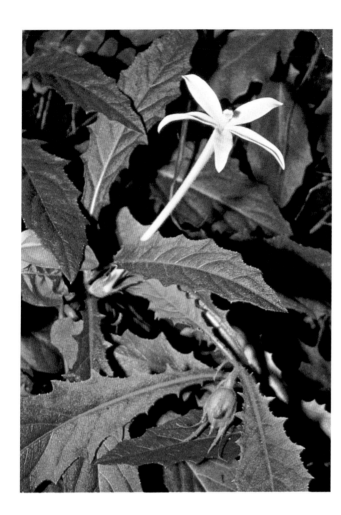

The star-of-Bethlehem plant contains a dangerous toxin that can be absorbed through intact skin. To be safe, never touch these plants. *(Art Whistler)*

# Toxin

All parts of the star-of-Bethlehem plant contain diphenyl lobelidiol, a central nervous system stimulant and extremely irritating alkaloid. This toxin can be absorbed through intact skin. All parts of this plant can also cause a skin rash.

# Traditional and Modern Uses

Traditional healers occasionally use this plant as herbal medicine, sometimes with fatal results. Using star-of-Bethlehem as a remedy is scientifically unproven and dangerous; it may result in death.

People sometimes smoke plants of this family in hopes of getting high. This, too, is potentially lethal.

# Incidence

Because of the instant toxic effects of even touching this plant, eating it by accident is rare. Poisonings are either from eating the plant in an attempt to get high or using the plant as an ingredient in herbal medicines. In 1997, the Hawaii Poison Center received one call from a person with star-of-Bethlehem exposure; in 1998 there were no calls.

On the mainland, an eight-year-old child died after having the juice of star-of-Bethlehem leaves applied to his head as medicine. The toxin apparently was absorbed through the skin.

# Signs and Symptoms

Star-of-Bethlehem sap in the eyes causes pain, tearing, redness, and swelling. Touching this plant can cause redness and a painful pins-and-needles sensation.

Generalized symptoms vary, depending on how much of the plant was absorbed through the skin or swallowed.

Eating star-of-Bethlehem often produces a metallic taste and profuse salivation. Stomach pain, nausea, and vomiting usually follow. Small doses speed up breathing; large doses slow it down.

Large-dose poisonings also cause euphoria, slow heart beat, high or low blood pressure, trembling, seizures, and paralysis.

 First Aid

Rinse eyes exposed to star-of-Bethlehem sap with tap water for 15 minutes. Scrub exposed skin immediately and thoroughly with soap and water. For continued pain and swelling, go to an emergency room. For symptoms of generalized poisoning, or any difficulty breathing, call 911. Take flowers, leaves, and a stem of the plant to the emergency room for identification.

## Advanced Medical Treatment

No specific antidote or diagnostic test exists for star-of-Bethlehem exposure. Decontaminate exposure areas; give charcoal for ingestions. Direct treatment at life support and relieving symptoms. Be prepared to treat seizures and hypotension and to protect the airway.

# TARO
## (Colocasia esculenta)

Taro is a food plant transported to Hawai'i by early Polynesian settlers. The main source of food in taro is the starch-filled, rootlike stem, called the corm, but the leaves, stems, and flowers are also edible when cooked.

People cultivate two types of taro: wet taro and dry taro. Wet taro grows along streams, in marshy areas, or in flooded terraces called lo'i. Dry taro grows in rainy upland areas, where rain is the only source of water.

Workers farm taro either by planting the suckers that sprout from the corm or by planting the crown with about 6 inches of stalk attached. Some varieties of taro bear seeds, which are also capable of producing new plants. The plants mature in 6 to 18 months, depending on the type of taro and the weather.

At least three hundred varieties of Hawaiian taro have been recorded, with distinctions based on size, shape, and color. The most familiar taro plants have smooth, heart-shaped leaves that grow a foot or two above the ground.

Most varieties of taro have calcium oxalate crystals throughout the plant. The amount varies with type. Some have almost none; others abound with crystals.

The calcium oxalate crystals in taro are rendered harmless by cooking.

## Toxin

All parts of most taro plants contain bundles of needlelike calcium oxalate crystals. Calcium oxalate is a nonabsorbable salt of oxalic acid, a colorless, crystalline, potentially poisonous

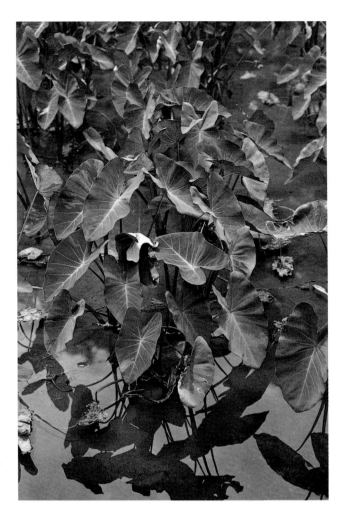

This type of taro is called wet taro because it is cultivated in a flooded terrace (the plants grow in standing water). Taro leaves and stems contain calcium oxalate, which can injure the mouth if eaten raw or undercooked. Cooking makes the crystals harmless. *(Susan Scott)*

organic acid found in many common food plants, such as spinach, rhubarb, tomatoes, grapes, and sweet potatoes. The human body produces its own oxalic acid. Some kidney stones contain calcium oxalate.

Whether eating calcium oxalate crystals is harmful depends on its concentration in a particular plant and on cooking methods. Some plants bearing this substance require no cooking, others require considerable cooking, and some cannot be made edible by any amount of cooking.

The amount of calcium oxalate in a plant varies greatly from plant to plant, and often even within the same plant.

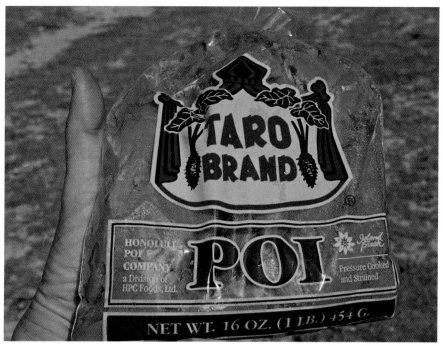

*Poi*, a food staple of ancient Hawaiians and still made today, is produced by cooking, pounding, and fermenting the rootlike stems, called corms. Taro corms contain calcium oxalate crystals but are rendered harmless by cooking. *(Susan Scott)*

A person must crush or chew the raw or undercooked leaf, flower, stem, or corm of taro to produce symptoms. The mechanical action causes special cells in the plant to inject the needle-sharp calcium oxalate crystals into the skin or mucosa. Chewing or crushing raw taro also causes the release of an enzyme that produces redness and swelling in the mouth.

Brief sucking on, or licking of, a leaf or flower usually is not harmful.

## Traditional and Modern Uses

Ancient Hawaiians used taro as food and medicine, and in ritual.

Most ancient Hawaiians preferred taro over sweet potatoes as their starch food. When taro was scarce, though, as in times of drought, it became the prized food of *ali'i*, or royalty.

The most important food made from taro was *poi*, a soft paste made of cooked taro root and water, then fermented. Taro leaves, stems, and flowers were also eaten. The Hawaiian name for boiled taro leaves, and for feast, is *lū'au*.

Ancient Hawaiians grew one type of taro just for medicine. Pieces of the corm of this variety, called *hoene*, were used as rectal suppositories to relieve constipation. Another type, *lauloa*, being low in calcium oxalate crystals, was grated raw and used in tonics for respiratory illnesses. Raw taro was also mixed with the ash of burned coconut meat and smeared in children's mouths to treat thrush. Today, people sometimes rub taro sap or leaf stalks onto rashes, cuts, or stings to aid healing. Ancient and modern uses of taro as a remedy are scientifically unproven and may be harmful.

The Hawaiian culture and the cultivation of taro were closely entwined. Only men could plant, harvest, cook, and mash taro. Women, though, were allowed to eat taro. Hawaiians sometimes placed taro plants on shrines, or altars, as offerings to certain gods.

# Incidence

Most people in Hawai'i know how to cook taro to avoid injuring their mouths with calcium oxalate crystals. Occasionally, though, the plant is undercooked, and the people eating it experience pain in the lips and mouth. In 1997, the Hawaii Poison Center received calls from twenty-three people exposed to raw or undercooked taro; in 1998, twelve people called. These numbers represent only a small fraction of the taro exposures experienced by Hawai'i residents and visitors.

# Signs and Symptoms

Raw taro sap or juice may cause a red, itching rash on the skin. Sap in the eyes may cause immediate pain, tearing, and sensitivity to light.

The main symptom of eating raw or undercooked calcium oxalate crystals is immediate pain followed by swelling of the lips, mouth, tongue, and throat. Some describe it as pins-and-needles pain. The victim often has excessive salivation, and blisters sometimes develop. Speaking may be difficult or impossible for up to two days. Swelling of the throat may make breathing difficult.

If a victim swallows any of this uncooked plant, vomiting and diarrhea may follow.

## First Aid

The pain and swelling from calcium oxalate crystals usually disappear slowly without special therapy.

Wash exposed skin immediately with soap and water. Try lifting embedded crystals with sticky tape. If the rash itches persistently, try 1 percent hydrocortisone cream 4 times a day, and 1 or 2 25-milligram diphenhydramine (Benadryl) tablets every 6 hours. Diphenhydramine may cause drowsiness: Do not drive, swim, or surf after taking this medication. Give children diphenhydramine syrup, following the dosage directions on the package.

For juice in the eye, rinse with large amounts of tap water for at least 15 minutes. Go to an emergency room for blurry vision, swelling, or prolonged pain.

If when tasting any part of this plant, even cooked, you feel a burning sensation, spit out all of the plant. Immediately rinse your mouth with water and spit that out, too. Try sucking on ice cubes to relieve pain, but do not swallow the ice water.

If any swelling occurs in the face, mouth, or throat, or if the victim has any difficulty breathing, call 911. Take leaves, stems, and roots of the plant to the emergency room for identification.

## Advanced Medical Treatment

No specific antidote or clinically useful diagnostic test exists for calcium oxalate rash, eye exposure, or ingestion. Most cases have only local symptoms, which usually respond to first aid treatment.

Calcium oxalate crystals do not dissolve in the digestive tract and therefore do not cause systemic poisoning. They can, however, cause severe burning pain, hematemesis, and bloody diarrhea.

Sap in the eyes may cause corneal abrasions or deposits of calcium oxalate crystals on the cornea. Irrigate thoroughly and examine with a slit lamp. Ocular steroids are unproven but are reasonable to try.

Pain medication may be necessary for both ocular and oral pain.

# NOTES AND REFERENCES

**Allamanda** *(Allamanda cathartica)*
*General References:* Baldwin (1979, 64; 1997, 37, 398); Harden and Arena (1974, 127–128); Kuck and Tongg (1958, 86); Lampe and McCann (1985, 27–28); Morton (1995, 147); Neal (1965, 687–688); "Plants—Dermatitis" (1992); "Plants—Gastrointestinal Irritants" (1992).

**Angel's Trumpet** *(Brugmansia x candida)*
*Notes:* 1. Coremans et al. (1994); 2. "Plants—Anticholinergic" (1995).

*General References:* Arnold (1968, 16, 17, 30); Baldwin (1979, 27–30; 1997, 139–141); Centers for Disease Control (1984; 1995a); Harden and Arena (1974, 137–139); Hassell and MacMillan (1995); Lampe and McCann (1985, 70–72); Morton (1995, 14); Neal (1965, 748–749); Wagner et al. (1990, 1252–1253).

**Anthurium** *(Anthurium* species)*
*General References:* Baldwin (1997, 52); Lampe and McCann (1985, 32–33); Neal (1965, 133–136); "Plants—Oxalates" (1996).

**Azalea** *(Rhododendron* species)*
*General References:* Baldwin (1979, 38, 85; 1997, 335); Harden and Arena (1974, 122, 124); Hodge (1996, 66); Lampe and McCann (1985, 142–143); Leikin and Paloucek (1998, 817); Neal (1965, 661); "Plants—Grayanotoxins" (1993).

**Be-Still Tree** *(Thevetia peruviana)*
*General References:* Arnold (1968, 8, 9); Baldwin (1979, 24–25; 1997, 381–382); "Digoxin Immune FAB" (1998); Harden and Arena (1974, 132–133); Haynes et al. (1985); Lampe and McCann (1985, 169–170); Morton (1995, 5–6); Neal (1965, 133–136); "Plants—Cardiac Glycosides" (1995); "Plants—Thevetia" (1992); Samal et al. (1992); Wagner et al. (1990, 205).

**Black-Eyed Susan** *(Abrus precatorius)*
*General References:* Arnold (1968, 11, 25); Baldwin (1979, 13; 1997, 13); Harden and Arena (1974, 81–83); Lampe and McCann (1985, 17); Morton (1995; 45–46); Neal (1965, 455); "Plants—Toxalbumins" (1992); Wagner et al. (1990, 638).

**Candlenut *(Kukui) (Aleurites moluccana)***
*General References:* Arnold (1968, 26); Baldwin (1979, 44–45; 1997, 30–31); Handy and Handy (1972, 228–231); Kepler (1998, 107–116); Krauss (1993, 101, 102, 103); Lampe and McCann (1985, 25–27); Morton (1995, 58); Neal (1965, 504–505); "Plants—Gastrointestinal Irritants" (1992); Wagner et al. (1990, 597–598); Whistler (1992a, 24, 49, 66, 79, 94, 110, 121; 1992b, 104; 1996, 71).

**Cassava *(Manihot esculenta)***
*General References:* Arnold (1968, 45); Baldwin (1979, 69–70; 1997, 251); Harden and Arena (1974, 118–119); Lampe and McCann (1985, 114–115); Neal (1965, 513–514); "Plants—Cyanogenic Glycosides" (1996).

**Castor Bean *(Ricinus communis)***
*General References:* Aplin and Eliseo (1997); Arnold (1968, 9, 10–11); Baldwin (1979, 20–21; 1997, 337–338); Harden and Arena (1974, 119–121); Lampe and McCann (1985, 144–145); Morton (1995; 53–54); Neal (1965, 509); "Plants—Toxalbumins" (1992); Wagner et al. (1990, 628–629).

**Cerbera *(Cerbera manghas)***
*General References:* Arnold (1968, 32); Baldwin (1979, 53; 1997, 103); "Digoxin Immune FAB" (1998); Neal (1965, 692–693); "Plants—Cardiac Glycosides" (1995).

**Cestrum *(Cestrum* species)**
*Notes:* 1. Coremans et al. (1994); 2. "Plants—Anticholinergic" (1995).

*General References:* Baldwin (1979, 56–57; 1997, 104–105); Lampe and McCann (1985, 53–54); Morton (1995; 23–24, 129–130); Neal (1965, 750–751); "Plants—Anticholinergic" (1995); "Plants—Solanine" (1996); Wagner et al. (1990, 1254–1255).

**Chinaberry *(Melia azedarach)***
*General References:* Arnold (1968, 46, 47); Baldwin (1979, 48–49; 1997, 253–254); Harden and Arena (1974, 100–101); Lampe and McCann (1985, 115–116); Morton (1995; 35–36); Neal (1965, 491–492); "Plants—Chinaberry" (1991); Wagner et al. (1990, 918).

**Crown Flower *(Calotropis gigantea)***
*General References:* Arnold (1949; 1968, 28, 29, 31, 39); Baldwin (1979, 55–56; 1997, 88–89); Crawford (1958); "Digoxin Immune FAB" (1998); Lampe and McCann (1985, 45); Neal (1965, 698–699); "Plants—Cardiac Glycosides" (1995); Wagner et al. (1990, 238); Wong (1949).

**Cup of Gold and Silver Cup (*Solandra* species)**
*Notes:* 1. Coremans et al. (1994); 2. "Plants—Anticholinergic" (1995).

*General References:* Baldwin (1979, 58–59; 1997, 359–360); Lampe and McCann (1985, 157); Neal (1965, 748); "Plants—Anticholinergic" (1995); "Plants—Solanine" (1996).

**Dumb Cane (*Dieffenbachia* species)**
*General References:* Arditti and Rodriguez (1982); Arnold (1968, 33); Baldwin (1979, 30–32; 1997, 145–146); Gardner (1994); Harden and Arena (1974, 48–50); Lampe and McCann (1985, 72–73); Morton (1995; 85–86); Neal (1965, 151–152); "Plants—Dieffenbachia" 1995).

**Elephant Ear (*Alocasia* and *Xanthosoma* species)**
*General References:* Arnold (1968, 22); Baldwin (1979, 64; 1997, 37, 398); Gutmanis (1976, 24, 26, 29); Krauss (1993, 16, 20, 103, 148); Kuck and Tongg (1958, 146); Lampe and McCann (1985, 29–30); McBride (1975, 27, 41, 79); Morton (1995; 88–92); Neal (1965, 156, 161–163); "Plants—Oxalates" (1996); Sohmer and Gustafson (1987, 17); Wagner et al. (1990, 1356); Whistler (1992a, 33).

**Foxglove *(Digitalis purpurea)***
*General References:* Arnold (1968, 33); Baldwin (1979, 63; 1997, 146–147); "Digoxin Immune FAB" (1998); Lampe and McCann (1985, 73–74); Neal (1965, 760); "Plants—Cardiac Glycosides," 1995).

**Gloriosa Lily *(Gloriosa superba)***
*General References:* Arnold (1968, 39); Baldwin (1979, 66; 1997, 185–186); Harden and Arena (1974, 44–46); Kuck and Tong (1958, 70); Lampe and McCann (1985, 85–86); Morton (1995, 37–38); Neal (1965, 190); "Plants—Colchicine" (1996).

**Hawaiian Poppy *(Argemone glauca)***
*General References:* Arnold (1968, 27); Baldwin (1979, 11–13; 1997, 59–60); Degener (1973, 164–166); Kepler (1998, 170–174); Krauss (1993, 102, 298); Neal (1965, 366–367); "Plants—Dermatitis" (1992); "Plants—Gastrointestinal Irritants" (1992); Wagner et al. (1990, 1004–1005); Whistler (1992a, 124–125).

**Hydrangea *(Hydrangea macrophylla)***
*General References:* Baldwin (1979, 39–40; 1997, 207); Harden and Arena (1974, 78–79); Lampe and McCann (1985, 94–95); Neal (1965, 381); "Plants—Cyanogenic Glycosides" (1996).

**Japanese Anemone *(Anemone hupehensis)***
*General References:* Baldwin (1979, 33; 1997, 50–51); Lampe and McCann (1985, 31–32); Neal (1965, 352); "Plants—Protoanemonin" (1992); Wagner et al. (1990, 1087).

**Jatropha *(Jatropha* species)**
*General References:* Arnold (1968, 11, 12, 45); Baldwin (1979, 16–20; 1997, 218); Harden and Arena (1974, 117–118); Ho (1960); Lampe and McCann (1985, 98–99); Morton (1995; 47–52); Neal (1965, 512); "Plants—Toxalbumins" (1992); Wagner et al. (1990, 621–623).

**Jimsonweed (*Datura* species)**
*Notes:* 1. Coremans et al. (1994); 2. "Plants—Anticholinergic" (1995).

*General References:* Arnold (1968, 17, 33); Baldwin (1979, 27–30; 1997, 139–141); Centers for Disease Control (1995b); Chan (1995); Harden and Arena (1974, 137–139); Lampe and McCann (1985, 70–72); Morton (1995, 16–18); Neal (1965, 750); Pereira and Nishioka (1994); "Plants—Anticholinergic" (1995); Salen et al. (1998); Vanderhoff and Mosser (1992); Wagner et al. (1990, 1255, 1257).

**Kāhili Flower and Silky Oak (*Grevillea* species)**
*Notes:* 1. Arnold (1941).

*General References:* Arnold (1968, 22, 40, 41); Baldwin (1979, 43–44; 1997, 189–190); Lampe and McCann (1985, 194); Morton (1995, 160–161); Neal (1965, 321); "Plants—Dermatitis" (1992); Wagner et al. (1990, 1086).

**Kava *(Piper methysticum)***
*Notes:* 1. Gutmanis (1976, 77); 2. "Newer Antidepressant Drugs Are Equally Effective" (1999); 3. Volz and Kieser (1997); Kinzler et al. (1991); Warncke (1995); 4. Anwar (1999); 5. Burlingame (1998); 6. Norton (1998); 7. Ngirasowei and Malani (1998); 8. Strahl et al. (1998).

*General References:* Baldwin (1979, 85; 1997, 308–309); Clark (1998); Degener (1973, 55, 98, 122, 152, 284, 286); Gutmanis (1976, 20, 24, 30, 33, 35); Handy and Handy (1972, 189–198); Krauss (1979, 1–2; 1993, 13, 22, 24, 35, 150); McBride (1975, 29); Neal (1965, 291–292); Wagner et al. (1990, 1036–1037); Whistler (1992a, 52, 69, 96, 112, 185; 1992b, 72–73; 1996, 59–60).

**Lantana *(Lantana camara)***
*Notes:* 1. Coremans et al. (1994); 2. "Plants—Anticholinergic" (1995).

*General References:* Baldwin (1979, 60–62; 1997, 229–230); Harden and Arena (1974, 135); Kuck and Tong (1958, 110); Lampe and

McCann (1985, 104); Morton (1995, 79–80); Neal (1965, 722); "Plants—Anticholinergic" (1995); "Plants—Lantana" (1997); Wagner et al. (1990, 1319–1320); Whistler (1992a, 165–166; 1992b, 96–97; 1995, 138).

### Mango (*Mangifera indica*)
*General References:* Arnold (1968, 22, 45); Baldwin (1979, 79; 1997, 250–251); Dang and Bell (1967); Morton (1995, 123–124); Neal (1965, 521–523); "Plants—Dermatitis" (1992); "Plants—Toxicodendrol" (1995); Wagner et al. (1990, 196–197); Whistler (1992a, 170; 1992b, 82; 1996, 75–76).

### Mushrooms (Agaricales)
*General References:* Arnold (1968, 23); Desjardin et al. (1998); "Mushrooms—Coprine" (1992); "Mushrooms—Cyclopeptides" (1998); "Mushrooms—Gastrointestinal" (1991); "Mushrooms—General" (1997); "Mushrooms—Hallucinogenic" (1997); "Mushrooms—Muscimol/Ibotenic Acid" (1994); "Mushrooms—Orellanine/Orelline" (1997); Smith (1980).

### Nightshade (*Solanum* species)
*Notes:* 1. Coremans et al. (1994); 2. "Plants—Anticholinergic" (1995).

*General References:* Arnold (1968, 53, 55); Baldwin (1979, 59, 73–74; 1997, 360–362); Gutmanis (1976, 24, 26, 27, 30, 35, 40, 45); Harden and Arena (1974, 141–145); Krauss (1993, 16, 67, 103, 294); Lampe and McCann (1985, 157–161); McBride (1975, 67); Morton (1995, 12, 30, 148); Neal (1965, 156, 742–744); "Plants—Anticholinergic" (1995); "Plants—Solanine" (1996); Sohmer and Gustafson (1987, 60–61); Wagner et al. (1990, 1267–1278); Whistler (1992a, 199–201; 1992b, 92; 1995, 129–132).

### Oleander (*Nerium oleander*)
*General References:* Arnold (1968, 13, 47); Baldwin (1979, 24; 1997, 269–270); "Digoxin Immune FAB" (1998); Harden and Arena (1974, 129–131); Haynes et al. (1985); Lampe and McCann (1985, 121–122); Morton (1995, 3–4); Neal (1965, 133–136); "Plants—Cardiac Glycosides" (1995); Safadi et al. (1995); Shumaik (1988).

### Pencil Plant, Crown of Thorns, Red Spurge, and Slipper Flower (*Euphorbia* and *Pedilanthus* species)
*General References:* Arnold (1968, 37–39); Baldwin (1979, 45–48; 1997, 169–172, 293–294); Harden and Arena (1974, 112–117, 119); Lampe and McCann (1985, 81–83, 128); Morton (1995, 104–107, 111–112, 113–114); Neal (1965, 519–520); "Plants—Dermatitis" (1992); "Plants—Euphorbiaceae" (1992); Wagner et al. (1990, 618).

**Periwinkle** *(Catharanthus roseus)*
*General References:* Baldwin (1979, 53; 1997, 100); Neal (1965, 689); "Vinblastine" (1992); "Vincristine" (1992); (Wagner et al. (1990, 215–216).

**Plumeria (*Plumeria* species)**
*General References:* Arnold (1968, 51); Baldwin (1979, 55; 1997, 312–313); Lampe and McCann (1985, 197); Neal (1965, 688); "Plants—Plumeria" (1998); Wagner et al. (1990, 213).

**Poinsettia** *(Euphorbia pulcherrima)*
*General References:* Arnold (1968, 17–19, 37, 39); Baldwin (1979, 45–48; 1997, 169–172); Harden and Arena (1974, 115); Krenzelok et al. (1996); Lampe and McCann (1985, 81–83); Morton (1995, 104–114); Neal (1965, 518); "Plants—Poinsettia" (1995); Wagner et al. (1990, 618).

**Pokeberry and Coral Berry (*Phytolacca* species and *Rivina humilis*)**
*General References:* Arnold (1968, 50, 51); Baldwin (1979, 35–36; 1997, 305, 338–339); Degener (1973, 103); Harden and Arena (1974, 69–73); Krauss (1993, 67); Lampe and McCann (1985, 133–134, 145–146); Morton (1995, 33–34, 149); Neal (1965, 339–340); "Plants—Pokeweed" (1992); Wagner et al. (1990, 618, 1015–1017).

**Star-of-Bethlehem** *(Hippobroma longiflora)*
*General References:* Arnold (1968, 43, 45); Baldwin (1979, 26–27; 1997, 232–233); Lampe and McCann (1985, 90–91); Neal (1965, 818); "Plants—Lobeline" (1992); Wagner et al. (1990, 472).

**Taro** *(Colocasia esculenta)*
*General References:* Arnold (1948; 1968, 22); Fung and Bushnell (1948); Handy and Handy (1972, 71–118); Ichiriu and Bushnell (1950); Kepler (1998, 203–210); Krauss (1993, 5–8); Neal (1965, 157–159); "Plants—Oxalates" (1996); Wagner et al. (1990, 1357); Wang (1983); Whistler (1992a, 113).

# REFERENCES CITED

Anwar, Yasmin. 1999. "Does '*Awa* Lack Punch Without Prayer?" *Honolulu Advertiser*, March 15, 1999, A1.

Aplin, Philip J., and Tony Eliseo. 1997. "Ingestion of Castor Oil Plant Seeds." *Medical Journal of Australia* 167 (September 1): 260–261.

Arditti, J., and E. Rodriguez. 1982. "Dieffenbachia: Uses, Abuses and Toxic Constituents." *Journal of Ethnopharmacology* 5:293–302.

Arnold, Harry L. 1941. "Kahili Flower *(Grevillea banksii)* Dermatitis." *Hawaii Medical Journal* 1 (September): 15–18.

———. 1944. *Poisonous Plants of Hawaii.* Honolulu: Tongg Publishing Co.; Tokyo: Charles E. Tuttle Co., 1968.

———. 1948. "Sour Poi is Safer than Sweet." *Hawaii Medical Journal* 7 (March–April): 313.

———. 1949 "Crownflower Keratonconjunctivitis—and Dermatitis?" *Hawaii Medical Journal* 8 (5): 354.

Baldwin, Roger E. 1979. *Hawaii's Poisonous Plants.* Hilo, Hawai'i: Petroglyph Press Ltd.

———. 1997. *Toxic Plant Index.* Rev. ed. University of Hawai'i. Computer Database. Honolulu: University of Hawai'i.

Burlingame, Burl. 1998. "Hawaii Looks to Cash in on Kava." *Honolulu Star-Bulletin*, September 7, A1, A8, C1.

Centers for Disease Control and Prevention, U.S. Public Health Service. 1984. "*Datura* Poisoning from Hamburger—Canada." *Morbidity and Mortality Weekly Report* 33 (20 May): 282–283.

———. 1995a. "Anticholinergic Poisoning Associated with an Herbal Tea—New York City, 1994." *Morbidity and Mortality Weekly Report* 44 (11 March): 193–195.

———. 1995b. "Jimson Weed Poisoning—Texas, New York, and California, 1994." *Morbidity and Mortality Weekly Report* 44 (3 January): 41–44.

Chan, Thomas. 1995. "Anticholinergic Poisoning Due to Chinese Herbal Medicines." *Vet Human Toxicol* 37 (2 April): 156–157.

Clark, Hugh. 1998. "Growers Banking on '*Awa* Boom." *Honolulu Star-Bulletin*, September 7.

Coremans, Peter, et al. 1994. "Anticholinergic Intoxication with Commercially Available Thorn Apple Tea." *Clinical Toxicology* 32 (May): 589–892.

Crawford, H. E. 1958. "Crown Flower Keratoconjunctivitis." *Hawaii Medical Journal* 17 (January–February): 244–245.

Dang, Richard, and Douglas B. Bell. 1967. "Anaphylactic Reaction to the Ingestion of Mango." *Hawaii Medical Journal* 27 (November–December): 149–150.

Degener, Otto. 1973. *Plants of Hawaii National Parks Illustrative of Plants and Customs of the South Seas.* Photo lithoprint reproduction. Michigan: Braun-Brumfield.

Desjardin, D. E., et al. 1998. "Agaricales of the Hawaiian Islands." Internet site <http://www.mycena.stsu.edu/hawaiian>.

"Digoxin Immune FAB." Revised in March 1998. Poisindex Toxicologic Managements 97. Database online. Denver: Micromedex, Inc., 1974–1988.

Fung, George, and Bushnell, O. A. 1948. "The Possible Role of Poi in the Epidemiology of Infectious Intestinal Diseases." *Hawaii Medical Journal* 7(4): 296–299.

Gardner, D. 1994. "Injury to the Oral Mucous Membranes Caused by the Common Houseplant." *Medical Oral Pathology* 78:631–633.

Gutmanis, June. 1976. *Kahuna Laʻau Lapaʻau. The Practice of Hawaiian Herbal Medicine.* ʻAiea, Hawaiʻi: Island Heritage Publishing.

Handy, Craighill E. S., and Elizabeth Green Handy. 1972. *Native Planters of Old Hawaii.* Honolulu: Bishop Museum Press.

Harden, James W., and Jay M. Arena. 1974. *Human Poisoning from Native and Cultivated Plants.* Durham, N.C.: Duke University Press.

Hassell, Harrison L., and Mary W. MacMillan. 1995. "Acute Anticholinergic Syndrome Following Ingestion of Angel's Trumpet Tea." *Hawaii Medical Journal* 54 (July): 669–670.

Haynes, Bruce E., et al. 1985. "Oleander Tea: Herbal Draught of Death." *Annals of Emergency Medicine* 14 (April): 350–353.

Ho, Richard K. B. 1960. "Acute Poisoning from the Ingestion of Seeds of *Jatropha curcas.*" *Hawaii Medical Journal* 19 (March–April): 421–423.

Hodge, Peggy Hickok. 1996. *Gardening in Hawaii.* Honolulu: Mutual Publishing.

Ichiriu, Edwin T., and B. S. Bushnell. 1950. "A Survey of Honolulu Restaurants for the Presence of Enteric Pathogens in Poi." *Hawaii Medical Journal* 9 (3): 166.

Kepler, Angela Kay. 1998. *Hawaiian Heritage Plants.* Honolulu: University of Hawai'i Press.

Kinzler, E., et al. 1991. "Wirksamkeit Eines Kava-Spezial-Extraktes bei Patienten mit Angst, Spannungs, und Erregungszustanden Nicht-Psychotischer Genese." *Arzneimittel-Forschung* 41: 584–588.

Krauss, Beatrice H. 1979. *Native Plants Used as Medicine in Hawaii.* Honolulu: Lyon Arboretum.

———. 1993. *Plants in Hawaiian Culture.* Honolulu: University of Hawai'i Press.

Krenzelok, Edward P., et al. 1996. "Poinsettia Exposures Have Good Outcomes . . . Just as We Thought." *American Journal of Emergency Medicine* 14 (November): 671–674.

Kuck, Loraine E., and Richard C. Tongg. 1958 (Tokyo.) *Hawaiian Flowers and Flowering Trees: A Guide to Tropical and Semitropical Flora.* Rutland, Vt.: Charles E. Tuttle Co.

Lampe, Kenneth F., and Mary Ann McCann. 1985. *AMA Handbook of Poisonous and Injurious Plants.* Chicago: American Medical Association.

Leikin, Jerrold B., and Frank P. Paloucek. 1998. *Poisoning and Toxicology Compendium.* Hudson, Oh.: Lexi-Comp, Inc.

McBride, L. R. 1975. *Practical Folk Medicine of Hawaii.* Hilo, Hawai'i: Petroglyph Press.

Morton, Julia F. 1995. *Plants Poisonous to People in Florida and Other Warm Areas.* Miami: Hallmark Press.

"Mushrooms—Coprine." Revised in October 1992. Poisindex Toxicologic Managements 98. Database online. Denver: Micromedex Inc., 1974–1998.

"Mushrooms—Cyclopeptides." Revised in March 1998. Poisindex Toxicologic Managements 98. Database online. Denver: Micromedex Inc., 1974–1998.

"Mushrooms—Gastrointestinal." Revised in February 1991. Poisindex Toxicologic Managements 98. Database online. Denver: Micromedex Inc., 1974–1998.

"Mushrooms—General." Revised in February 1997. Poisindex Toxicologic Managements 97. Database online. Denver: Micromedex Inc., 1974–1998.

"Mushrooms—Hallucinogenic." Revised in April 1997. Poisindex Toxicologic Managements 98. Database online. Denver: Micromedex Inc., 1974–1998.

"Mushrooms—Muscimol/Ibotenic Acid." Revised in January 1994. Poisindex Toxicologic Managements 98. Database online. Denver: Micromedex Inc., 1974–1998.

"Mushrooms—Orellanine/Orelline." Revised in February 1997. Poisindex Toxicologic Managements 98. Database online. Denver: Micromedex Inc., 1974–1998.

Neal, Marie C. 1965. *In Gardens of Hawaii.* Honolulu: Bishop Museum Press.

"Newer Antidepressant Drugs Are Equally Effective as Older-Generation Drug Treatments." March 18, 1999. Press Release. Agency for Health Care Policy and Research, Rockville, Md. <http:/www.ahcpr.gov/news/press/pr1999/deprespr.htm>

Ngirasowei, Janice, and Joji Malani. 1998. "The Relationship Between Sakau (Kava) and Gastritis." *Pacific Health Dialog* 5 (September): 266–268.

Norton, Scott A. 1998. "Herbal Medicines in Hawaii from Tradition to Convention." *Hawaii Medical Journal* 57 (January): 382–385.

Pereira, Carlos Alberto L., and Sérgio de A. Nishioka. 1994. "Poisoning by the Use of Datura Leaves in a Homemade Toothpaste." *Clinical Toxicology* 32(3): 329–331.

"Plants—Anticholinergic." Revised in December 1995. Poisindex Toxicologic Managements 97. Database online. Denver: Micromedex Inc., 1974–1998.

"Plants—Cardiac Glycosides." Revised in August 1995. Poisindex Toxicologic Managements 97. Database online. Denver: Micromedex Inc., 1974–1998.

"Plants—Chinaberry." November 1991. Poisindex Toxicologic Managements 97. Database online. Denver: Micromedex Inc., 1974–1998.

"Plants—Colchicine." Revised in April 1996. Poisindex Toxicologic Managements 97. Database online. Denver: Micromedex Inc., 1974–1998.

"Plants—Cyanogenic Glycosides." Revised in June 1996. Poisindex Toxicologic Managements 97. Database online. Denver: Micromedex Inc., 1974–1998.

"Plants—Dermatitis." Revised in January 1992. Poisindex Toxicologic Managements 97. Database online. Denver: Micromedex Inc., 1974–1998.

"Plants—Dieffenbachia." Revised in December 1995. Poisindex Toxicologic Managements 97. Database online. Denver: Micromedex Inc., 1974–1998.

"Plants—Euphorbiaceae." Revised in October 1992. Poisindex Toxicologic Managements 97. Database online. Denver: Micromedex Inc., 1974–1998.

"Plants—Gastrointestinal Irritants." Revised in January 1992. Poisindex Toxicologic Managements 97. Database online. Denver: Micromedex Inc., 1974–1998.

"Plants—Grayanotoxins." Revised in May 1993. Poisindex Toxicologic Managements 97. Database online. Denver: Micromedex Inc., 1974–1998.

"Plants—Lantana." Revised in October 1997. Poisindex Toxicologic Managements 97. Database online. Denver: Micromedex Inc., 1974–1998.

"Plants—Lobeline." Revised in August 1992. Poisindex Toxicologic Managements 97. Database online. Denver: Micromedex Inc., 1974–1998.

"Plants—Oxalates." Revised in June 1996. Poisindex Toxicologic Managements 97. Database online. Denver: Micromedex Inc., 1974–1998.

"Plants–Plumeria." 1998. Poisindex Toxicologic Managements 97. Database online. Denver: Micromedex Inc., 1974–1998.

"Plants—Poinsettia." Revised in December 1995. Poisindex Toxicologic Managements 97. Database online. Denver: Micromedex Inc., 1974–1998.

"Plants—Pokeweed." Revised in October 1992. Poisindex Toxicologic Managements 97. Database online. Denver: Micromedex Inc., 1974–1998.

"Plants—Protoanemonin." Revised in June 1992. Poisindex Toxicologic Managements 97. Database online. Denver: Micromedex Inc., 1974–1998.

"Plants—Solanine." Revised in June 1996. Poisindex Toxicologic Managements 97. Database online. Denver: Micromedex Inc., 1974–1998.

"Plants—Thevetia." Revised in July 1992. Poisindex Toxicologic Managements 97. Database online. Denver: Micromedex Inc., 1974–1998.

"Plants—Toxalbumins." Revised in February 1992. Poisindex Toxicologic Managements 97. Database online. Denver: Micromedex Inc., 1974–1998.

"Plants—Toxicodendrol." Revised in August 1995. Poisindex Toxicologic Managements 97. Database online. Denver: Micromedex Inc., 1974–1998.

Safadi, Rifaat, et al. 1995. "Beneficial Effect of Digoxin-Specific FAB Antibody Fragments in Oleander Intoxication." *Archives of Internal Medicine.* 155 (October): 2121–2125.

Salen, P. N., et al. 1998. "Clinical and Epidemiological Characteristics of a Jimsonweed Epidemic." *Annals of Emergency Medicine* 32 (3 September): 54.

Samal, K. K., et al. 1992. "Clinico-Pathological Study of *Thevetia peruviana* (Yellow Oleander) Poisoning." *Journal of Wilderness Medicine* 3:382–386.

Shumaik, G. M. 1988. "Oleander Poisoning: Treatment with Digoxin-Specific FAB Antibody Fragments." *Annals of Emergency Medicine* 17 (July): 732.

Smith, C. W. 1980. "Mushroom Poisoning in *Chlorophyllum molybdites* in Hawaii." *Hawaii Medical Journal* 39 (January): 13–14.

Sohmer, S. H., and R. Gustafson. 1987. *Plants and Flowers of Hawaii.* Honolulu: University of Hawai'i Press.

Strahl, S., et al. 1998. "Necrotizing Hepatitis after Taking Herbal Remedies." *Dtsch Med Wochenschr* 123 (November): 1410–1414.

Vanderhoff, Bruce T., and Kevin H. Mosser. 1992. "Jimson Weed: Management of Anticholinergic Plant Ingestion." *American Family Physician* 46 (August): 526–530.

"Vinblastine." Revised in September 1992. Poisindex Toxicologic Managements 97. Database online. Denver: Micromedex Inc., 1974–1998.

"Vincristine." Revised in July 1992. Poisindex Toxicologic Managements 97. Database online. Denver: Micromedex Inc., 1974–1998.

Volz, H. P., and M. Kieser. 1997. "Kava-Kava Extract WS 1490 versus Placebo in Anxiety Disorders—A Randomized Placebo-Controlled 25-Week Outpatient Trial." *Pharmacopsychiatry* 30:1–5.

Wagner, Warren L., et al. 1990. *Manual of the Flowering Plants in Hawaii.* Vol. 1. Honolulu: University of Hawai'i Press and Bishop Museum Press.

Wang, Jaw-Kai. 1983. *Taro.* Honolulu: University of Hawai'i Press.

Warncke, G. 1995. "Psychosomatische Dysfunktionen im Weiblichen Klimakterium. Klinische Wirksamkeit und Vertraglichkeit von Kava-Extrakt WS 1490." *Forschr. Med.* 109:119–122.

Whistler, Arthur W. 1992a. *Polynesian Herbal Medicine.* Honolulu: National Botanical Garden.

————. 1992b. *Tongan Herbal Medicine.* Honolulu: Isle Botanica; distributed by University of Hawai'i Press.

————. 1995. *Wayside Plants of the Islands.* Honolulu: Isle Botanica.

————. 1996. *Samoan Herbal Medicine.* Honolulu: Isle Botanica.

Wong, Wayne W. 1949. "Keratonconjunctivitis Due to Crownflower." *Hawaii Medical Journal* 8 (May–June): 339–341.

# Index

For classic symptoms of plant exposures, see Quick Guide to Hawai'i's Poisonous Plants, pp. xvi–xvii. For plant relationships, see Families of Poisonous Plants in Hawai'i, pp. xiii–xv.

# ABOUT THE AUTHORS

Susan Scott has written a weekly column, "Oceanwatch," for the *Honolulu Star-Bulletin* since 1987 and is the author of three books about Hawai'i's environment: *Oceanwatcher: An Above-Water Guide to Hawaii's Marine Animals, Plants and Animals of Hawai'i,* and *Exploring Hanauma Bay.* A registered nurse since 1974, Scott earned a bachelor's degree in biology from the University of Hawai'i in 1985.

In 1997, Scott and Thomas wrote as co-authors *All Stings Considered: First Aid and Medical Treatment of Hawaii's Marine Injuries.* The book spurred their interest in other nature-related injuries in Hawai'i, leading to this book and its companion volume, *Pests of Paradise: First Aid and Medical Treatment of Injuries from Hawai'i's Animals.*

Besides being co-authors, Scott and Thomas are diving buddies, trekking partners, and a volunteer doctor-nurse team for the Aloha Medical Mission. They have been exploring Hawai'i together since they moved to the Islands in 1983.

Craig Thomas is a practicing physician, board certified in family practice and in emergency medicine. He is president of Hawaii Emergency Physicians Associated, Inc. (HEPA), a physician group that provides medical coverage for the emergency departments of Castle Medical Center, Wahiawa General Hospital, Hilo Medical Center, and North Hawaii Community Hospital. Thomas is medical director for the Honolulu Fire Department and the Honolulu Police Department, and is a member of the clinical faculty at the John A. Burns School of Medicine, University of Hawai'i.

Thomas has practiced emergency medicine in Hawai'i since 1983. He has hiked extensively in Hawai'i and throughout the world. Busy as he is, Thomas is still a person who stops frequently to smell the flowers. After writing this book, he now knows which ones are poisonous.